I Dre‌
Auti‌

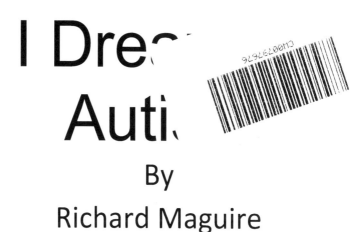

By
Richard Maguire

Published by A PENN PR 2014

Buckinghamshire, United Kingdom

www.anniepenn.co.uk

www.autismlivetraining.com

Prologue

Richard has impressed me both as a person and as a writer. In meeting and getting to know him I discovered someone who has had to learn about the rules of being a human almost from scratch... acquiring them the hard way, diligently writing about this journey for us all to see.

His book is a testament to the heart and spirit of people who have autism - a subject that is often overlooked by the media and some professionals working in this area.

I find it significant that most people are interested in the 'autistic mind' but clearly Richard reminds us of the importance of his heart which feels both pleasure and suffering like any other. Following his heart, along with his wish to understand and be understood, Richard used his intellect to map out a way of living that he uses and refines every day in being within his world. Fortunately, his propensity for sharing has allowed him to develop and offer this gift to the many clients he works with and those reading this book.

Not everything we read here is straightforward or easy to understand and that is wonderfully deliberate. Richard makes an audience wrestle with trials and tribulations to understand his own experiences and that of others like him.

This is not an autobiography in the traditional sense but a sharing of a state of mind - an invitation to both understand and communicate. It is also a subtle offer to many neruo-typical readers that through the course of absorbing his story they begin to change both personally and, if necessary, professionally.

Dr Emilios Lemoniatis, MBBS BSc AKC MRCPsych
Consultant Child and Adolescent Psychiatrist at The Tavistock and Portman NHS Foundation Trust, London

Testimonials

Richard Maguire is one of the most inspirational people I've had the privilege to know. Diagnosed with Asperger's syndrome as an adult, many might consider Richard to be 'mildly affected' by autism. He has extraordinary skills as a trainer, a wonderful sense of humour, drives a car, holds down a job and is married with a son. On the face of it, his life does not seem to have been overly troubled by autism.

This outward appearance belies the extreme nature of the difficulties he faces and needs to overcome daily in order to succeed. Richard is a highly valued core member of our Autistic Training Team at Autism Oxford and I hope that his book reaches into the hearts and minds of those who can make a difference to people who, like him, live as actors on life's neuro-typical stage.

Kathy Erangey, BPhil PE Cert ASC
Managing Director - Autism Oxford

Of all the autobiographies by people with autism that I've read, 'I Dream in Autism' is different. It isn't just an account of the author's (often painful) experiences but takes one right into the centre of what it feels like to be on the autistic spectrum. From the beginning Richard invites the reader into his head, to share his sensory distortions and goes on, 'Are we sitting uncomfortably? Then we are ready to begin.'

My attention was grabbed. The ensuing text is long, meandering and at the same time, absolutely riveting. Personally, I find his technical descriptions of his cameras fascinating, especially where he is able to relate these to his ability to crystallise how he feels. Holding emotions through a viewfinder was a new idea to me and there were many others. Every teacher should read this book.

I Dream in Autism tells us just how misleading some current ideas about autism are:

People with autism do not feel emotion. Wrong!

People with autism do not have a sense of humour. Wrong!

Children with autism are 'lazy', 'naughty', stupid'. Wrong!

That 'being quiet' necessarily indicates improved behaviour rather than deeper withdrawal. Wrong. (I wrote this in a report about a child a few weeks ago before reading this book. I was told she was more tolerant of children kicking the patterns she was assembling on the floor and this indicated an improvement.)

Phoebe Caldwell, DSc

For my wife Julie
And my son Joshua
I love you both more than words can say

Inspiration

You cannot teach a man anything, you can only help him find it within himself.

Galileo Galiei

I never teach my pupils, I only attempt to provide the conditions in which they can learn.

Albert Einstein

Outside of school, though, we were often defined by our disabilities. We were 'handicapped' a bit like a species. Often when people have a disability, it's the disability that other people see rather than all the other abilities that coexist with their particular difficulty. It's why we talk about people being 'disabled' rather than having a disability.

One of the reasons that people are branded by their disability is that the dominant conception of ability is so narrow. But the limitations of this conception affect everyone in education, not just those with 'special needs'.

These days, anyone whose real strengths lie outside the restricted field of academic work can find being at school a dispiriting experience and emerge from it wondering if they have any significant aptitudes at all.

Sir Ken Robinson

A Simple Trust - quiet, simple, unspoken, understood... void of complexity, free of ambiguity, all social cues removed. Spoken in the silence. Take time and be still, practice serenity in simplicity. This is really all that is needed to come along side autistic people. It helps with distressed neuro typical people also.

Richard Maguire

Not quite alphabetical… not quite in order… not quite
conforming… just like autism

If you would like to work with Richard Maguire, please visit
www.autismlivetraining.com

For other information please call: A Penn PR 07742937154
www.anniepenn.co.uk

Introduction – Autism, It's Life But Not As We Know It...

I have wanted to write a book on autism for many years. I am autistic and have worked with autistic people for decades. Being autistic and focused means I have sought to understand autism and how the autistic life is lived. The answer is 'differently'. We piece together sounds, sights and feelings in real-time. Autistic development, senses and processing are unique to each autistic individual. We develop along paths quite distinct to each one of us. Yet, in all of this, there are crossed paths and ways of learning. Many people who are not autistic can sense the life of autism and become very good at communicating with autistic people. I have worked with and trained hundreds of these people.

I use my own experiences in this book as they are the ones I can describe most fully. It also means I need not be concerned about confidentiality. Every view is my own. I have written about selected times and themes, along with specific sections on employment and observations from the perspective of how things evolve for me, and the significant factors people overlook that are important to us autistics.

Each chapter is as it is - some long, some short. I have written my book in this way to replicate the fragmentation in the autistic mind. As you read, you will pick up a common theme: there is no order. Start at the back, front or middle – it's your choice. I wanted to give you that freedom of choice as it conveys how I approach thought. The content is shaped by what people find useful in the training, education and family work I do as an autistic counsellor and training consultant. Often, in my written prose, I will seek to paint a picture with words that describes how precise and confusing the autistic life is. I have spent over thirty years working with learning disabled people suffering from many syndromes, but specialised in autism mentoring, as I am defined by my autism... and my results.

In my work, I will always place central emphasis on promoting a positive culture around autism and building up relationships that allows autistic adults to feel valued and happy about themselves. I also help neuro typical (what you would describe as 'normal') colleagues to deepen their understanding and empathy for autistic service users. When this compassion and way of working is internalised, neuro typical people can appreciate that developing relationships with autistic individuals and their close/extended families, friends, employers – you name it... is a happy experience with constructive outcomes.

The autistic life I know best is my own and it's my trusted resource in the work I do. I knew nothing of autism until 1985 when I worked with an autistic person. It clicked right there and then - I recognised how similar we were and accepted it.

Autism was not widely understood when I was a child in the mid-1960s but as you read this book you will see how it has become the foundations of my work for over thirty years. Autism has its own life, feel and energy. To know autism is to know this life. Nowadays, I am delighted to celebrate my idioms, meltdowns, stimming (repetitive stimulating such as leg jerking or frantic walking), OCD (obsessive compulsive disorder), erratic behaviour and many other wonderful nuances that maketh me. I have almost died because of them. But, thankfully, I was one of the lucky ones that survived.

I have spent years writing this book in order to tell you how public and private organisations use my experience and findings to help others gain success and triumph over this inelegant mantle.

So, let's get started... Firstly, I need to put you in my head. I want you to notice the noises of the world around you – whether you are on a train or watching television or tucked up in bed, it doesn't matter. Just pay attention to every single noise in your immediate vicinity. Next, you need to feel the impurities from the breath of strangers on your skin – it doesn't have to be anyone around you but think back and obsess about those you walked past earlier today. Did you wince or wash it off? Good – almost there. Now I need you to glance at the light source above you (single bulb or vast expanse of sky) and shy away from its intensity. And finally, start to feel anxious in every moment. Okay, job done.

Are we sitting uncomfortably? Then I can begin.

In a world that overloads us with sound and information, we autistic people see detail with piercing clarity. People ask us about these details and assume we understand the whole, but in actual fact we are still working on the whole while seeing the minute details – sometimes we can't see past those details. Problems arise when people assume we see everything this clearly, but a lot of life is a big mystery and we need time to make sense of it. Autistic individuals have a deep thought process that operates very slowly and steadily. It starts with unravelling the details to 'get there'. Neuro typical people make these connections almost instantly, leaving our actions to be mistaken for rudeness.

Growing up with Enigma is the first chapter in this book. It gives a personal view on my developmental years with autism. Other autistic lives will differ to mine but we share the same anxieties and uneven progress. Interestingly enough, when young, we autistics quickly learn to 'fake it' and act exactly like the people we see around us. Or we become passive hoping not to get noticed. Anxiety always kicks in, and we want to run away with the 'fight or flight' emotions that give us so much pain. Often it's a combination of these things at various times.

The way through varies for each one of us but we need to be able to process life, communicate and feel good about who we are. That requires a sensitive approach and an amount of knowledge on autism. I do not profess to have the answers or claim any cures for behaviour reasoning, I simply tell my tale. Go on into the book with the spirit of being autistic – rejoice in repetition, understand and feel intense passion for emotional and intellectual output. Explore and gain insights for use in a life centred on being different and if you want to know about the title the answer is in there too.

11

Growing Up With An Enigma

Enigma: an inexplicable occurrence or situation

Inexplicable occurrences and situations have been my life's setting. I have a store of information in my head. Holding this information is a constant, necessary weight. Every day, I trawl through masses of sensory information and memories to seek a plan for tackling the day ahead. Life makes more sense as years pass, and gradually I have put together many mental forms and templates for understanding it – enabling how I can act in the world.

Interpretation of details, making mental templates, building up a mind-matrix of understandings and actions are something I help a lot of autistic people to do. With these in place, an autistic person is on the way to what I call **'initiation'** (the point at which there is enough of a matrix for them to make their way in life effectively). Until that point, we are often stuck in an overload of processing intricate details without any means of direction.

I have initiated my life and seen other autistic people initiate. It's like witnessing the launch of a space rocket, seeing them experience a blast of confidence shot deep into their core. A lifetime of details come together into a discernible and useable matrix and the person is off in a purposeful direction quickly, decisively and with a good deal of happiness.

The next thing to facilitate is a series of further matrixes to deal with things when life goes wrong - being let down by people and how to modify a matrix to take changed circumstances into account.

Here is how I started out. I was born autistic. My earliest memories are of enigmatic situations, behaviours and communications. Life was, and still is, a series of confusing details that are not easy to put together into a whole or even to recognise as details needing connection. It's like having a head full of raw experiences without interpretation or understanding. As an adult, I have amassed a large framework of understandings

13

against which to check the sensory details of life. I use this knowledge to build up concepts and to see life as a whole.

But as a child, life was a frightening and incomprehensible procession of details. People had an expectation that I could make sense of this and react, but I had no idea - I had to work it out in the long dark nights when the house was still and no one interrupted me. Life, when everyone was awake, made no sense.

I remember being invited to a birthday party (late 1960's), in a neighbour's house along with my baby sister and Mum. Lots of children were there and it was fun, noisy, energetic and confusing. I was distracted from the party by the hexagonal paving slabs outside, the tessellating pattern of blue and black on the living room carpet and the contrast between carpet and parquet flooring in the dining room. The children wanted me to play, but the only game I understood was 'What time is it Mr Wolf?', a simple game involving walking gingerly towards Paul, who was being Mr Wolf, and pretending to freeze when he turned to look at us. If he saw movement we were out of the game. The winner had to get to the finish line and safely out of the wolf's way.

I knew this game because it had simple rules. Normally I was advised, criticised and chastised at parties. However, I do recall some words from the adults, 'Go on Richard' or 'Go now Richard'. What they did not know was that I really did want to go, but the G-Plan furniture and the configuration of colour tone on the carpet captured my attention. And I loved the way the patterns moved from different viewpoints - they always fitted. The social necessity of playing Mr Wolf became lost in the noise as I admired the designs on the floor and felt captivated by the profile of the dining table legs. No one else did this but me. Why were adults saying 'Come on!' or 'Go now Richard!'? I just couldn't work it out.

Thankfully, nothing unpleasant happened, such as me being told off, and the party carried on, a distant rumble of moments and expectations. I got through it well enough and enjoyed myself. The food was great - I could sit and chill on my own with a colourful paper plate full of party food. I could be an observer, feeling the atmosphere of the party. I could perceive fun and happiness if I didn't have to move - that would have overloaded my processing, meaning I could not sense the party to enjoy it. Adults showed signs that they accepted my stillness. It was okay to be still when eating. I had no idea why, it just worked.

Before we moved to Aylesbury on my fourth birthday, I remember being confused and not sure of what was going on at my own party. What was my role? I was told it was my birthday. Great! I would get presents and people would make a fuss of me. I remember feeling happy about this and seeing lots of food. Then the children came. I had already met some of them. However, I could not recognise or place most of them as I don't remember faces. My mother expressed concern that I did not know who each of the children were.

I remember being given presents and becoming confused with a feeling of being overloaded. Most of my interactions with the other children were distant and I went very quiet. They soon lost interest in me and went to do something else. That day I had lots of attention, but I felt unable to deal with it. Knowing what to say did not come into this since I had no idea I needed to say anything at all and a very good idea that something wasn't right. My head reeled with strain from children moving in my peripheral vision. I recognised the noise as speech, but could not comprehend words and meanings when directed at me. Speech went everywhere like a ringing babble. I knew when I was being spoken to sometimes though, as my mother would tell me that someone had come to say hello. She also did this when I was given presents.

I had no concept of dealing with receiving gifts. I remember clearly unwrapping one present - it was two Matchbox cars. I loved Matchbox cars. Whoever bought it for me knew what I liked and I was very pleased. But two cars? I felt greedy and that confused me. A present was singular but here I was holding two. I remember looking at them thinking I should not accept double gifts. I offered one of the toy cars to the boy who had given them to me feeling happy with my action and assuming that he would be happy too, but he didn't seem to know what to do, nor did I. My mum spoke to me and said I was going to keep both cars they were my present. I got the impression I had done something wrong.

I knew I did things wrong and felt disapproval from people many times. I was getting used to this and the embarrassment of regularly making mistakes. I felt pain at my party as I knew things were going badly. They always did when groups of people were around. On reflection, I can see my child-self had no grasp of how to behave at a party or the rules and behaviours that went with it. This party cemented for me an expectation that life was a series of embarrassing experiences to be endured.

I was constantly being told I was old enough to know better, followed by expressions of disapproval, sanctions and punishments... and, at school, bullying. Yet I simply did not have the social ability to process society's expectations. From that day, I learned to be passive. It led to fewer chastisements and less embarrassment. This would set the standard for most of the rest of my life. I decided to be like wallpaper and not to be social since the consequence of social gatherings hurt. I craved a pain-free life and to reach that basic goal I endured a lonely, longing existence.

I have come across many autistic adults who grew up like me. A retrenchment into a small interior world is preferable to one of social interaction and the inevitable hurt that accompanies each attempt. But this can be overcome. It takes time and a lot of confidence-building, guidance and honest appraisal. Quiet behaviour from an autistic child is not always good - check the context. This retreat into oneself builds up an uncontainable pressure of anger, anxiety, frustration and masses of things that do not get said. Explosive meltdowns will happen, maybe years later.

Existing in a passive fashion meant I could put lots of chastisements away. I disengaged and led an internal life. It also meant I did not learn much socially and acquired the label 'quiet'. Many years later, when my wife reintroduced me to someone who knew me at school she was amazed saying that I used to be so silent that she was concerned about me. I was not all right, I was in pain and did not want to attract more by risking interactions with people. I was also out of practice at having relationships with anyone outside of my immediate family. And I had no any idea what to do about it.

My fourth birthday party was a turning point - the start of my withdrawal. I did not have birthday parties after that. Birthdays had presents and a birthday meal with my family, but this was a treat instead of a party. My parents knew I was not good at parties. I did not have enough friends to make a party anyway; I had no friends to invite.

The following September I started school, which brought a whole new host of horrors. Children ignored or bullied me - they certainly didn't want to be my friend. I learned from some children that even if they wanted to be friends with me they would avoid the opportunity to be seen in my company. I was untouchable as a friend and made so unpopular that no one would come out and say they liked me. With the joint acceptance of life being a roundabout of confusing experiences and withdrawal being my modus operandi I set off into a sad and quiet childhood.

Unsurprisingly, the distance between me and interacting with other people deepened over the years until it was impossible to hope for a normal friend. I really wanted friends like everyone else and to be sociable. I knew I was interesting, sincere and friendly but realised nobody else cared about me.

Feeling unable to communicate on any meaningful level with most people intensified daily. Instead, I looked forward to family social events, but when they happened I found them confusing too. Demands of expectation overwhelmed me as I tried to get a handle on recognising a face, matching that up with their name, avoiding looking at the weave on their knitted jumper, being blinded by flickering kitchen lights, other family members asking questions at the same time. Hearing a tutting noise and being told to leave the room. Shame on me.

I felt lost, unable to know where I would fit in, and continued to seek out quiet spaces away from the masses of people. I had no openings for conversation and that has still not changed. If anyone did approach me to talk I could try to engage in my way and get deep into a subject that interested me before noticing that my relative had stopped listening. Then I would try to talk about something else, getting back to the original subject later thinking it was not finished. But they weren't bothered about odd little me - they were so mercurial in their attention span that I lost all means of understanding what was happening.

Eventually, I would feel as if I had failed and withdraw into my quiet world away from the noise and social prickle of festive or family gatherings. Being out of it was painful, lonely and unfulfilling - as was being in it. I was criticised for my social faux pas (committed frequently, causing embarrassment and drawing down social opprobrium). I really did not understand what was happening, or what to do. I couldn't read other people's body language or learn from them how to operate in a social context. Acceptable behaviours became incomprehensible blurs, resulting in people being surprised, shocked or critical of me.

Occasionally, I saw that my idiosyncratic conduct amused people and that's when I realised they were not being nice. Their own ignorance of my autistic state meant they were burdened with me and trying their best to cope with a boy who seemed different to the point of distastefulness. I was just someone to be dealt with or taught a lesson. I hated being laughed at and was often called a freak, dippy, strange, dilly daydream and stupid. These are adults and family. I believed every word they said. I felt their looks of distain and knew I was being tolerated but not liked. Inside me the pain was intense as I struggled with being different to other children, and with the fact that I was not liked or accepted.

Aware that I could not behave or use language like a 'normal' person, I began employing the only accessible human behaviour models I could – characters in TV programmes. My first and last observational study was the cast of Scooby Doo. I started identifying myself with Shaggy and Scooby. Velma appealed to me because of her intelligence and rigorous ways of working things out, just like my ways of thinking. Eventually, I married a woman very like Velma. My wife Julie only speaks after a lot of thought and makes logical sense when she does. So, as a boy, I tried copying these TV characters, but with little success, returning to being very quiet and avoiding the company of others.

I have never been able to learn much from 'live people' as they give off too much to process. This made getting on with people when I was young very hard. I recall frequently losing ground in the social arena via a sickening and out of control process. I just could not keep up. I tried ever so hard, but just could not digest the information overload, and that frightened me. I did not want to be like this, yet no matter how I tried, I lost more ground, becoming extensively out of touch. I did not ask for this to happen. I wanted to be 'normal' like everyone else.

Another watershed moment was at the house of one of my mother's colleagues - 'Auntie Nell' as I knew her. There was a gathering… I think she had retired. Other teachers (my mother was a teacher) were there, along with my family. The downstairs of Nell's half-timbered cottage was full of people, hot and noisy. Groups of adults were moving around the building with noise coming out of them – greeting me and shaking my hand – but as I was unable to carry on a conversation, they left me alone.

My family got on with talking to guests and I was left looking at the old oak beams and the open fire, reflecting on how I was no good at these kind of gatherings. I was also sure now that I was a very boring person. This was how I understood my lack of social ability. I was boring and no good to anyone - people saw this and left me alone. Their minds and motives were a conundrum to me and I carried these convictions with me for decades.

I was convinced that I was a dull young man that no one wanted to be burdened with. A large amount of hope left me and I pondered my future. How lonely would I be? How could I live this life of isolation? What of any ambitions? I did not have any belief back then that I was intelligent and could turn my hand to build wonderful things. I just stood in that room, knowing I was growing up and wondering how would I get anywhere in life by being alone, boring, and in pain.

While thinking through this bleak vision, I noticed that Nell's dog didn't come near me. I usually attracted animals and knew this dog well, but as feeling of poor self-worth settled on my seven-year-old shoulders I became inconsolable with silent grief - even the dog didn't want me. I felt wooden and dead inside.

As the days and months passed, I became more concerned about what was happening. I seemed to be drifting away from people. I knew that they did not find me cute anymore, which had been my failsafe as a young child, getting me out of lots of difficulties. My parents had different expectations of me now. I had observed growth and reflected on the stages of life – disturbed and dejected children have the space to recognize this. They are different and told it is wrong. I saw my peers moving into new ventures that I was unable to follow without a mental framework for comprehending and enabling normal living. I observed well, I could commentate, but I neither understood nor coped in company.

The enigmas in life grew as I grew. I hoped to learn how to get on with other people and thought if I applied myself well enough maybe I could catch up. This did not happen. I had no basis for identifying what was happening to me and why I was different. If only there was a diagnosis of high functioning autism, dyspraxia and dyslexia in the 1970s... Instead, I was just told I was naughty and maladjusted. People said I did not try hard enough. I heard the word 'lazy' far too often and it crushed my spirit. They did not know I tried so very hard to survive every single day without being told off. Slowly and surely their own framework for approval pushed me into a broken mould. I became convinced that 'lazy' referred to my inability to develop. Life became a round of criticisms and being ignored. I had very few openings for love and fun.

I grew up in a typical suburban Home Counties scenario. English middle-class life involves a measure of anxiety about being better than the neighbours. Lots of this involves status management (dinner parties, driving the right car, having a higher than normal profile job) and high academic expectations of your children. It's a stupid culture, dictated by frightened people forced to compete using table manners and out-of-date ethics, usually steeped in Victorian morals. Everyone lived behind the façade of perfection. All had a path to follow and it was expected that the children would become respectable members of society – doctors, lawyers, teachers etc.

My parents discussed their children at every opportunity. What would we become? The question was brought out at social and family gatherings by other acquaintances too and then raised lots more at home for good measure. Expectation is laced on children. I saw parents discussing their children's development - saying what they had achieved and what they would go on to do as adults. It seemed to me that we were valued for what we did and what we would do. Simply finding a role to enjoy and be happy was not enough. Achievements mattered, in exams most of all. Our futures and earning potential were debated and aligned with the world of work from when we were young.

I watched mothers vie for a higher status by acknowledging (politely) their offsprings' achievements. We did not seem to be valued for who we were and it incensed me. We were held up and paraded at social gatherings - looking well dressed, well behaved and intellectually capable of appreciating the 'finer things' in life - not pop music or pop culture. We all loved pop music but parents quashed this in polite company. And when it came to discussing me, my parents had little to talk about... I was a quiet, underachieving oddity. No musical prowess, no academic achievements.

I was certainly not neat! I hated wearing posh clothes due to my intensive sensory needs. When I could be scrubbed up for social events, I was depressed and surly, hating it all and hating the clothes I was told to wear. I would usually back up into a corner wanting to go home or get out on my bicycle. I use to analyse middle class life, hating the snobbery, pretence and value put on things that had no intrinsic worth. I wanted to be valued for being me. Some part of me would have liked to gain achievements for my parents to brag about, but I reckon they were as troubled as me. I am sure they had no idea why their obviously intelligent son achieved so little, got so grumpy and withdrew in every social situation.

Of course, I felt pressured to do better, and became convinced that this was the way to develop as a person. I thought that doing things made people interesting and popular. As I couldn't read the social skills that really made people affable, I modelled an idea that being good at music, cultural activities and exam success made people fun, interesting and socially acceptable. This set my social development back years, intensifying feelings of loneliness. I could not talk about music, culture and academic things. I could talk about bicycles but no one else thought this was important.

It was a grey existence being on the margins of middle class life. I wore a grey school uniform and hated it. (I still do.) I looked at my school jumper and decided my existence was just as grey. I had no place to get a purchase on life. No point of fun and acceptance. I lived in a dreary, fog like, drizzle-filled life. Lonely, very lonely.

Don't feel sorry for me, though. This is not a whinge. This is an open window into the mind of a child who was as frightened of himself as he was of the fear he coaxed from others by surviving in the only way he knew. There was some comfort gained from being young. I knew I would be cared for and could still get off the hook by 'not knowing any better'. I also knew I was growing up. Ever year took me closer to adulthood.

The pain grew greater with the awareness that I would reach physical maturity without the wherewithal to get on in adult life. I was behind my contemporaries in understanding the twists and turns of culture. I also knew I was not stupid but somehow felt unable to deploy my intelligence. I often observed other intelligent children in my classes at school showing their brilliance and getting respect for this. They were able to be bright and popular. I was bright and bullied or ignored - both hurt in different ways.

The spiral of being unable to understand why I was losing out continued. I just knew I was missing out on everything. I could see others gain popularity and tried to catch up, but fell flat. I knew where I wanted to get to, but the way there made no sense. More than that, I could get no understanding of 'normality' to materialise in my consciousness – I had no framework to operate by, because of all the interferences from other avenues. Sensory overload cramped my hearing and sight; anxiety fed my awkward mannerisms. I was aware I behaved in one way and my peers another. Believe me, I tried to be normal, whatever that was, but my head, heart and soul could not comprehend what to do. More than that, I had a total block. I spent ages trying to work out what was happening, unable to rationalise anything internally and sick with worry. The only information I had to go on was feedback from other people – and it was not good feedback.

At school I was called slow, lazy and stupid. I was often excluded from school events – by being ostracised or by missing out because of the inevitable detentions. The teachers were okay, but not really interested in helping me. They viewed me as eccentric and dealt with me in a reasonable way. The trouble was that the other children would pick up on my differences and attempt to speed me up in class whenever my attention wandered. This led to cruel songs and cutting verbal abuse - they had a handle on me that they could use to wind me up.

One taunt was to chant to the tune of Tulips from Amsterdam, which started 'It's true, I know, Richard's so slow'. This was sung repeatedly in the playground. Not one teacher stopped it. I reacted with incredible anger that caused them to sing it more. In class, I would see other areas of enquiry related to subjects and

I Dream In Autism

drop my focus on the lesson - my head full up of interest and questions. Or I would be infuriated by my classmates and their taunts.

At home my parents expressed concern over my lack of progress, despite my obvious intelligence. Laziness was an obvious answer given their ignorance of my condition. All in all, I received negative and despondent feedback from my parents. I contemplated their negativity and became convinced that I actually was bad, lazy and no good to anyone. I also thought about occasions like the gathering at Auntie Nell's house and the loss of hope they engendered. I was unable to see any hope for my future and saw myself sliding out of human society. This trapped me into a sense of worthlessness and hopelessness.

Birthdays came and went, quietly without much in the way of celebration – I still did not have friends to attend parties. I felt at each birthday that I, too, was slipping away, out of life and into oblivion. Looking into my future was painful as it reflected more agony - an adult me, rejected, overlooked and finding no love or fulfilment. I felt pain from being an intelligent and talented person with no possibility of enjoyment from all the potential I carried. I faced a future of entrapment in a dull life lived between loneliness and rejection.

I knew a route to happiness existed… somewhere. I did not know the means of being happy, or what it would feel like, as my own existence was a sort of grey limbo and I did what I needed to do to get by. But I had a small grain of hope within me, an undefined hope that things would get better. I hadn't a clue how, but I needed to hope.

Decades later I do have happiness, friends and family. Today I work with autistic people who are living with the pain I had. And I tell them 'There is hope'. An autistic person lost in the wilderness of enigma and separation from all that is life-affirming wants the same thing - someone to believe in them. Someone who can communicate and help them learn in the autistic way where happiness is to be found.

So much of happiness in society is learned the neuro typical way. This leaves the autistic person sitting on an island of incomprehension and emotional distance. A useful way of learning is through instruction, practice and un-judgemental feedback. We so often need a brick of a person who will not criticise us and is able to see our beauty and talent. In a one-to-one relationship, with structured learning, we can practise life, have fun doing it and find fulfilment.

We really do need the same things as neuro typical people. We share the same humanity and need of relationships. Inside we are full of love. That love is normally shown and expressed in the majority – so neuro typical culture is our difficulty. We live alongside and do not comprehend the workings of this culture. We appear distant, maybe aloof. This impression is a misreading of our incomprehension of the enigma that is neuro typical life. We bounce off it and are unable to get through the layers between us - communication, love and affirming rapport. We pace, cry, hurt and despair on the outside of human life, receiving disapproving messages and rejection. This becomes the central hurting place of incomprehension and break in relationships.

Lots of the autistic life is lived like this, surrounded by people who have different ways of approaching life to us. We set of into the same situations, then see and get interested in different things and different ways of seeing life. Other people appear out of a moving fog of humanity, form, noise and colour. It becomes apparent at times that they want to interact with us but we don't notice the cues and signs that they want to interact – hence we do not respond as they expect us to. We are racking our brains for the right things to do and say. They become baffled by our actions, turning the interaction into an awkward moment that is internally fraught for the autistic person. We seek an exit strategy or simply cannot proceed. It all goes wrong.

The trouble is that we like the person who approached us and wanted to get on well with them. We are often sad that things do not go well and cannot work out how to put things right. We try to get out and about without experiencing these difficult interactions. Going places can become easier if we have prepared for it beforehand, and have had our confidence built to cope with an awareness of the unexpected at all times.

Cultures that surround us are interesting and incredible. When embarking on my teens I was spellbound and fascinated by the youth and pop culture around me. I understood it in an autistic way - I was a complete outsider wanting in on this exciting music and fashion. I just did not have a clue where to begin. This showed in the way I dressed and what I did. What I really wanted were guidelines and logical explanations of these cultures and how I could access them – just like the physical and mental frameworks I build for clients today.

I also wanted to know how to dance, as I enjoy feeling the music resonating deep down in my soul, but have no idea how to connect physically with this, so avoided discos for fear of being made fun of for not knowing what to do. I had plenty of taunting outside of social events and knew it would be intensified if I went out with other teenagers.

I recall one evening when a local disco was on. My sister went. Dad and I waited in the car and I so wanted to go in, but stayed sitting, as if frozen in my seat. I knew if I could understand what was going on and get in I would be happy, but didn't have a clue about how to tackle the situation. The culture among my contemporaries had moved on in a way and with a speed I could not have foreseen. I remember my dad saying that I should try the disco. He said there were lots of people my own age in there and I would make friends. I replied that I did not know what to do. My sister told me my uncoordinated attempt to dance was unacceptable and I would have to learn properly. She was right and I knew it. I said to my dad that I would go to discos and parties if I could learn what to do, and by that I meant being taught in a logical way. He said that if I went in I would learn (this would be okay for a non-autistic neuro typical person who knew the rules). No one was aware of my autism back in 1980 and we drove home in silence. I felt deeply grieved for the missed opportunity, but couldn't face the ridicule of judgmental individuals.

I also wanted a girlfriend and realised this was impossible – I was not cool. Girls said they would never go out with me. I accepted this and lived my closed life. How to get a girlfriend was beyond me, yet I knew I had so much love to share. I wanted the closeness of this sort of relationship, and ached to feel cherished by someone. Because I had not been out with a girl it was often assumed I was homosexual. I endured hate taunts that gave me insights into the suffering gay people tolerate because of their sexuality.

This targeted animosity helped me to develop a strong sense of empathy for minority causes – me being one. I have carried this sense of justice on into adult life. In this respect, being autistic helps a lot. I am not bothered about getting attacked for standing up for people who are vulnerable. I believe in equality amongst all people - this is logical and right in my autistic mind. I do not comprehend the need to define others as different and to loathe them for it. I feel the hurt and know just how horrid it is to be put down for something, anything that is different from the norm.

I had no idea about the politics used to conduct life. I frequently watched television news and wondered why people lied – saying one thing but meaning another. I also did not understand why people were not literal – they never did what they said they would do, or they acted in a way that was inconsistent with a belief they supposedly held. I also could not get to grips with the viewpoints of different newspapers. I thought that if there is an event then there is one truth and the public need to know that truth. I did not understand the nature of biased reporting. Being an autistic thinker means I took everyone at his or her word, becoming confused and annoyed when they failed to deliver promises.

I still put everything people say to me into a framework, but today I factor in the probability that they may not say what they mean. I need to work out various scenarios based on the likelihoods of alternative interpretations. This involves a huge amount of mental processing. Being in social situations can be tiring and I regularly need to remove myself for moments of restorative brain space. I have cottoned on to the fact that neuro typical people communicate with more than words and learned how to spot the thousands of non-verbal means of communication people use.

I watched myself on a CCTV recording at work once and became struck by my absence of body language. I was like a statue compared to the other two people in the film. I studied non-verbal communication and how it augments or changes the meaning of the words people use and became astute at recognising these actions. I never study in the way 'normal' people do it. I use everyday opportunities allowing for observation, logic and contemplation before cross-referencing it on my database of social signals to empathise and interpret these signals. 'Normal' people simply smile and start a conversation.

At times in my life, I have used this cultural crossover from autistic to normal to achieve aims in negotiations. Being autistic means I have a good poker face - I will give nothing away. I used to be a union steward and this technique helped immensely. I could unnerve people opposed to me by not playing the game and standing up for what is right. Sometimes people would remark on how hard I negotiated – not giving an inch. Inside I knew I was just being autistic and playing straight down the middle.

I was keen to leave my teen years behind in one sense, but knew I was not getting anywhere in life and needed a mentor – which would never happen. Nowadays, I am mentor to many young adults and see the same situations developing, only here we handle them with objectives and targets that build up self-esteem to allow exploration of conversation. Imagine that! Having a conversation and being able to process it for long enough to feel valued!

As I grew up, I did find a rare bit of company - I used to inhabit the bicycle sheds at break times to escape the bullies. This was far enough away from the playground and the politics going on there.

Interesting and unusual students would gather in the cycle sheds talking about all sorts of subjects. For a precious moment I was accepted as I fixed their bicycles. I am an expert at bike maintenance and worked out that I could get on with people one-to-one by offering a skill they wanted. I also knew a lot about people from observing them. I didn't talk much and was my usual introverted self but people love a captive audience. They thrive in talking about themselves - some would open up to me with their deepest thoughts and issues.

I started to find out more about what was going on than the chatty people in the playground. As I repaired inner tubes and straightened spokes or oiled chains, no one felt the need to put on a front. They seemed to realise that I did not merit such things. However, back in the classroom they would completely blank me in front of their friends - it was bad for their ego to be associated with me. I had one particularly good cycle shed visitor - a girl called Clare. She was not like lots of the other girls. She had a kindly countenance, genuine warmth and was in no way superficial.

Clare was a real help in my loneliest teenage times. I knew I would never be accepted by the 'group' but I could see a friendly face in Clare. I lost touch with her after school and only found out where she was immediately before she moved to New Zealand. I would have loved to get to know her and catch up on life in between. I hope you are happy Clare.

It's strange, but a lot of people memorably close to me are in reality as far away as New Zealand. I often do not have the required matrix of conversational procedures for contacting them. They may be close but I lack the cognitive set up to make contact. There are still a lot of gaps in my matrixes. Sometimes I am too tired to repair them, or act, once I have made the cognitive connections and practiced the words. I may be a few feet from you and wholly incapable of making contact.

I muddle through explanations of situations to myself after they happen. When I do get an understanding, I will try and commit it to memory and place it within my mental matrix for next time. At the same time I need many sub-matrixes for every permutation on that situation, as I am aware it will not be exactly the same next time. When the next time does appear, I am able to trawl my memory to find a cognitive match for the situation – making further adaptations for the here and now. If the situation moves too fast, it may have a new variable I did not foresee or I may experience sensory overloaded and my cognitive abilities will break down.

If I am overloaded, I am unable to process anything. Sensory breakdown is the most frequent reason I cannot interact and I stumble at the first step. At these times I am quiet and withdrawn, or I go into what I call 'slug mode' and crawl along quietly on some old routines trying to maintain a presence for a time at least. Slug mode is horrid, I hurt a lot and feel pretty horrid and want to go away and cry, but instead I sweat it out pretending I am okay.

I do not think anyone who knows me understands how hard daily interactions are and how much information I can't gather from their mannerisms, or how broken down my senses are through overload and the feeling of anxiety that causes. Life is disconcerting, broken up and largely incomprehensible, only able to be solved later in the quiet when I can do my processing and work out what is going on.

Being A Visual Thinker And Using Words

My life is lived in films - I run them in my head, long ones and short ones. They are often run in quick succession and sometimes it's as if they are running concurrently. All information taken in is converted to visuals to be processed and worked on. Once I am clear with their content and meaning they are filed and fitted into the totality of my memory bank. I can overlay these films onto reality, like a head-up display. It takes a lot of processing so normally they play in my head. Words follow the actions at key points in the memory cinema.

Repetition is important - thoughts are rehearsed into my memory and words added where necessary, altered a little sometimes on each repetition. Every thought is modelled, run and re-run. I insert variables and cross-reference, link up with other thoughts, make connections and synthesise new thoughts into new visual scenarios. These too can be run to model and test how they work. Thoughts tumble over and over, as if they are in a great, turning drum. New ones are inserted, others displaced and some forgotten.

I must know the inner workings of everything I see and do, building visual models for as much as I can. When I was a child I did this for everything in my life. I recall back in the late 1960's examining the floor, sills and mechanics of my dad's car. I wanted to know if it was made from solid metal, and if the floor was a single sheet of metal or if it had further layers and structures underneath.

I did not think the floor would be strong enough if it were a single sheet of thin metal and I worked out the pressed channels in the floor gave three dimensions and stiffness. I wondered why the sills and box sections were hollow and went to find out why. This lead me on to learning about tubes and that a structure with three dimensions that is hollow in the middle is as stiff as one that is solid and of the same dimensions, but much lighter.

Today, forty years later, if I can see under a car I will stop to look. I am still transfixed by structures and how they deal with forces. I am also interested in how better materials, pressing techniques and computer aided design have resulted in fewer panels and joins in every generation of cars. I like finding out about high strength steels and where they go in relation to car body shells. I walk to work past a car dealer where transporters are parked outside regularly, allowing me to stop and examine the assembly process. Every time I do this, I recall being a four-year-old examining my dad's MK II Cortina, tapping the vehicle doors, looking underneath and making the first models of cars in my head.

From my dad's car, I learned how to analyse and visualise a mechanism's inner components. Then I moved on to discover which parts of the structure were load bearing and which were not. From there I graduated to observing the development of everything - houses, ships, the planet, the freezer, my bicycle, our garden fence, the structures in wood, trees and smaller plants... then bones, crystals and micro assembly, then grass and plant stems, model aeroplanes, real aeroplanes, tractors with their load bearing transmissions, pens, cakes, eggs, clothing fibres and weaves, glue and glued joints, tyres, furniture, ceilings and roof beams, so on and so forth.

Throughout the years of my childhood, I built up a library of visual understandings of structures. As far back as I can remember I would project and rotate visual models of things in my head like a computer simulation. I can subject them to different forces and model their behaviour, plastic deformity and failure modes.

Even today, when I buy a car, I have to inspect every joint in its entirety. I take parts off and remove the trim to see inside. I must see all the fragments of engineering connected together in the vehicle and read a manual so I can analyse the parts in the engine and gearbox that I am physically not able to see. I know exactly how the engine in my current car is made – it's a clever design using lots of aluminium and as little metal as possible. I have examined every piece of webbing cast into the block, making it stiff and light. I rev up the engine to feel the forces going through it. There is a resonance in the crankshaft and cam chains that I am sure was not intended when the engine was designed, but is a product of a lack of stiffness, causing cam chains and tensioners to fail.

I build up a visual model of all the lines of force and resonance in the engine and transmission. I have watched all sorts of lubricant fluids operate to understand their effectiveness. I researched the preferred oils used by mechanics, watched liquids flowing, studied shafts and bearings, dismantled oil pumps, checked out the oil return system, assessed the air spaces in the engine, looked at engine cross sections. At any speed I can visually replicate what is going on in my car engine, including the oil flow, combustion and gas flow. I have checked out the exhaust and assessed what it is doing in relation to back pressure, gas management, resonance, sound insulation, silencing and releasing gases to the air. It's hard work driving and knowing all this is going on.

I have spent hours studying tyre manufacture and the formations in tyres, the banding and layering of a tyre. I have examined all the areas of tyres and explored what they do including their variant degrees of contribution to the suspension on my car and how forces are managed. Movement, compliance in the bushes, arcs of movement, passive steering, geometry, sound insulation and strengths, stiffness and thicknesses of materials.

As I drive, I visually model my car working. It took me years to visually model valve timing and phases on a four cylinder engine but I was obsessed and use all this visualisation every time I drive. Its hard mental work, but I can always get the best out of my car. The level of detail I undertake to discover and log these details is much more than I have written here but I think you can get the idea. All this effort to drive a K11 Nissan Micra! This is how an autistic person operates – remember that when you give one a lift or ask about their interests.

When I buy another car, I will be studying it in exactly the same way. My car is old with a moon-shot-mileage clocked up and I want to hold on to it as long as possible, I have it mapped in my mind though many images, some with sound. Before the Micra I drove Citroen 2CVs, five of them. I mapped them all out in my mind too with the same intricate effort and am still a member of the owners' club.

I took great interested in understanding all the materials used in my house and endeavoured to research how it all works together. I have seen under the floors, in the roof, behind the plaster and studied how our humble Victorian home is built straight onto levelled-off clay (with no foundations!). Lime mortar makes the building resilient and flexible - its strength being in elasticity and absorption of forces. The house moves and breathes in a similar way to trees. This building has stood for over 130 years, yet nothing in its design has failed and I know why (in minute detail). I can rotate, up end and examine our house in my mind in flawless, mentally catalogued detail. I wonder how 'normal' people view their houses.

Then on to my bicycles. I know their assembly in even more painstaking detail. I examine tubes, joints, machining, spokes, drive train efficiency, materials, lubrication and the synergy of the whole bicycle in relation to the rider. Don't forget, I spent a lot of time on my own as a young person with no friends. This was a way of coping with my unusual life.

One of my bicycles folds in half - a Brompton. It's delightfully clever and efficient. I can see that the hinges are at points of maximum strength and folding practicality. All its manufacturing arrangements are designed with great simplicity, strength, ease of use and durability. Another in my collection is a Moulton bicycle with triangulated and separable space frame, small wheels and full suspension. No part of the Moulton's structure is redundant. It is massively stiff and very efficient. The suspension is designed for road use and works at high frequencies, allowing high pressure tyres to be efficient with a comfortable ride. I study the frame and can see all the ways it deals with forces and loads. I see and feel the whole machine in action from any angle in my mind when I ride it.

The third bicycle is a Bob Jackson - a traditional layout diamond framed machine with large wheels. It is unique, bespoke and finished beautifully. Again there is a synergy between the machine and me; I feel so alive and am eager to get on with going anywhere. You would need to be a bicycle enthusiast to understand what the Reynolds 531 ST tube set is and what this does for ride quality and feel, but trust me, it works like nothing else; the bike is like a living organism when in use. I know how the tubes are cold drawn. They have no seams or inconsistencies and the ideal tube structure, bringing out the best properties of steel.

Then I have an old Raleigh Lenton an elegantly simple sports touring bicycle from 1950. A good old friend. Yes, these machines became my steadfast companions.

I have Brooks' leather saddles on all four bicycles. I researched and learned about the composition of the stitch and properties of skin, which has been tanned and made into saddles. I know how these saddles are broken-in by my movements and how they are shaped to my own body and joint peculiarities. I took time to see just how my muscles and skeleton work in relation to the bicycles and how different types of saddles help with posture or positioning.

I live in a world of vivid colour and form. All thoughts, emotions and senses are translated and processed in form and colours first, words second. Words are my second language, I think and process everything in pictures and colours with their accompanying tastes, using words alongside pictures to discern and describe finer details. This use of words helps me to anchor memories and make plans. I have wondered if this is because words are not natural, and the process of making, ordering and using them requires thought, helping to tease things out. Pinning up visuals with words, like notices on a corkboard, kind of works. The words are immobile yet the visuals they hold move with life, carrying meaning, feelings and love.

Learning to use words was hard and still requires much preparation, thought and effort. I try to stock up on the words needed for each day the night before. There are ways of conveying precise meanings that do not use words, but words are the prefered way of communicating used by people everywhere. To be taken seriously and viewed as intelligent I must use spoken words. Written ones are even harder.

Using words requires a five-stage process. Words are:

Heard

Translated into visuals

Processed and understood

Translated back to words

Spoken

I cannot speak an image. I wish I could. Words are rehearsed and put into memory singly or in phrases, many thousands of them. Visuals pass over them, picking up the words, editing them mentally and speaking them as sentences while the film runs in my mind and soul. Words are pins, things precise points, pieces of exact meaning. None is abstract. Abstracts, feelings, emotions, thoughts and my soul are all in pictures.

I find words frustratingly lacking in visual meaning. I remember sitting an oral examination for English at school. I surprised the examiners by saying that I thought written works were boring at first sight and they need to be worked on through reading to uncover their splendour and interest. The examiners did not expect that answer and awarded me a good mark for the critique I gave of writing as an artform. I reflected on that exam for decades; now I know I was commenting from the viewpoint of a visual autistic thinker. I can take in visual art naturally and appreciate it from first sight. When connecting with written art I must work on it.

In the process of engaging with something that is such hard work I think I get more from the art when I have finally comprehended it. That could be the work of minutes to years, analysing, interpreting and processing. I have also developed a way of being very eloquent with words, written or spoken. This eloquence is the result of a lifetime of struggle with words in any form. I think that what did not come easily has become something I have worked hard on and have applied myself to. As a result, I give thoughtful and hard won expression in the form of words. Every word counts and has been crafted and used with thought, I have to wrestle with articulation and language and I think I have developed a deep respect for words.

It's not that I like words or using them. I use them well because I must and the process is hard. So, I have written a book. I have wanted to write a book since I was small. I have been looking for subject, material and technique until I realised it was already inside my head. I just needed to tell the world how I felt. I wrote about feeling trapped by non-autistic people and their judgement so that families with autistic relatives and friends can start to understand.

For decades I have listened to BBC Radio 4 - programmes such as *Open Book, A Good Read* and *Book Club*. I can rarely read a book in one sitting because of the effort and memory needed to log the information in my own unique system – it can get too much and too complex, but I read bits of books seeking what I can from them. I had years of reading as I retreated into myself and my world without social interaction.

BBC Radio 4 is a medium I use to channel information into picture building - insights about books and writing, listening to authors as they describe the writing process. Describing narrative, their characters and where their stories take them while being written are valued help in the struggle to express my work in normal written form. I am grappling with voice and narrative as I listen, eager to capture my stories in the right words. These stories that are stored in my head as films have been shared with published authors, who say there are good stories that could be written well.

So I hope I am doing some justice to my message of hope. I still do not have a 'gestalt' (over all understanding), for narrating a story, however I am working on this and have been for decades. I desperately want to tell adults and children stories of life and all that does not make sense. Because it does make sense when explored through the characters. Well, sort of sense...

I believe human lives are not finished while we live, nor should a story be finished. My stories are steeped in the lives of the people I work with and focus on offering them help from someone that has been there - me. The characters can live and engage with what does and does not work for them and maybe it only works as a shadow of what it could be. The characters develop even though they barely exist. They stay alive and their life is just that... life, given that it is the expression where they find themselves that matters.

Many plots and settings are dark and lack meaning. If the significance of their tale is found it still doesn't explain much and leaves them unfulfilled. In the darkness, characters have to be creative, dig in, gain traction for survival and carry on using their main resource - hope. The stories progress to points in life where a hard won improvement or juncture is met. And that's it – arrival, with or without understanding, then life goes on.

The theme I explore is being human and having a happy fulfilling existence – that is powerful and creative in itself, and even if all influence over life or a grip on reality slips for a time, the living of life matters. Living life is good even if it hurts or ceases to make sense. The resolve to live is central to my stories. A lot of the explorations are of my autistic world and realising that with planning and hope there is an opportunity to be content - I must engage, try and trust in myself. That is good, living is good, and life must be worked at. Just like writing, and the innovative workings out of understanding life.

This, for me, makes words a source of more life, better life and a life that can be communicated and grown into new relationships over time. The protagonists in my stories face goodness knows what every day to stay in the human race (and in doing this they must choose life) - even if they do not understand it or see a purpose. Like my childhood and teenage years, by persisting, they live life as they grow until for a fortunate few it becomes a good thing. My job is to walk with them and keep the characters developing with enough confidence to bring about success.

I am a visual thinker forced to use words. Thank you BBC for giving me words and the life that goes with them. Most days I listen to Radio 4 to do what I call 'mining for words'. I refresh and add to my word library in my visual notice board, ready for use in the right context.

The use of words did not come easily. Firstly, I copied what people said, but that didn't work well as I had no idea of how to issue words correctly. The words belonged to the person speaking them and I felt they should remain in that context. It is unusual when a child uses adult forms of words but no one told me that. I found adults easier to listen to, as they normally spoke slowly and in lower pitches. Children moved too much, spoke fast and lacked the arrangement that adults used in speech. It is often observed that autistic children sound like adults when speaking. Learning words from adults is easier as they are more precise and predictable - they have a better command of meaning and a richer vocabulary.

As explained, I spend a lot of time building matrixes to form a basis for every part of life. This is the same with words. Conversation for me requires comprehensive and structured matrixes, plus a lot of side loops containing understandings for subtexts and deviations from the main subject. That's a lot of work, so to help I pre-prepare practise and memorise thousands of sentences and sound bites (yes really), keeping them stored for use so I can appear to be speaking spontaneously. When I learned that people do not give you the time to prepare words I decided to have a bank of scenarios readily available. That involves hours of preparation for every day and uses a lot of memory. I get tired in conversation very quickly.

I can remember sometime in the mid 1970s wondering why I couldn't keep up in conversations and why I got caught out a lot with no words to speak. Back then, I had no idea I produced speech differently and was told I was the same as everyone else but a bit more stupid. I was also described as slow and lazy until I believed them. Top tip – don't say any of these things to an autistic child or even imply they are sub-standard, as your words will be taken into adulthood and held close in the form of destroyed self-esteem. Autistics take you at your word – we literally take the words from your mouth and believe them. We have to work hard trying to cope with everyday life and those negative comments are often at the root of suicide attempts later in life. Think about that before jumping in with criticism.

So, back we go to the mid 1970s. I knew that I was slow with words of any sort because of the elements of my condition, yet I was unaware of any condition. People around me could box me in with words. Deep in my soul I had words, but was paralyzed to argue. The person I knew who was fast and comprehensive with words was my mother, so I listened intently with an aim to be quicker than her. She was a safe bet to study as she was around me a lot, and if I modelled my vocabulary on her eloquence I would get misunderstood and bullied less. I applied myself to the understanding of conversations, words, their placement and use, then recorded conversations in my head and analysed them.

I also listened to hours of BBC Radio 4, wondering why people did not believe the words politicians used, aware that the commentators dug deeper for the real meanings. The *Today* programme showed that people did not say what they meant - especially politicians. However, it would be decades before I learned that people did this in all areas of life - seeking to deceive others for unknown reasons. Being a truth speaker, I learned those lessons the hard way. I understood that politicians lied, but being true to my autistic nature I did not generalise that insight.

Teaching people to generalise forms a large part of the mentoring work I do. We autistics do not generalise naturally. Instead we like to use many sub-rules explaining the real sub-text inconsistencies with life and communication. That means carrying lots of rules about everything and its variables, then accessing a mental database of rules quickly in every social situation in order to respond.

I must have been about ten or eleven when I thought I had mastered speech well enough to hold my own. That worked reasonably well with adults interested in a subject, but not so well in general talking or at school, but it was a milestone in building interaction skills.

In this section, have written about the use of words - only spoken or written words. Intonation and expression are still mysteries to me. I know people use them, but all I hear are voices going up and down. Intonation and emphasis carries no meaning for me. I act on words alone. This is the autistic way of receiving and using language. I have been trying all my life to make visual connections to tone and emphasis in speech, and had a few attempts based around mouth shapes, observing when people use emphasis, but these are incomplete and tenuous. I do not have a cognitive handle on tone and emphasis, I look for signs people are doing this – an audible clue. I am a visual thinker and can only understand things to any depth through visuals.

Please don't try to interpret the monotone speech of autistic people in any way as you will learn nothing about our mood or feelings from the way we deliver words. Many of us, me included, have learned to copy intonation and emphasis because we have learned it's expected in some situations. We are acting out an alien form of communication - for your benefit. We realise non-autistic people want and expect these things. We find people are nicer to us when we do this and believe what we are saying. It's like speaking a foreign language at the same time as speaking English.

Between learning from my mum and Radio 4, I built up a mental lexicon and could read complicated texts. At aged eleven I read books for sixteen-year-olds, which was all down to consciously collecting and learning words.

I like words for their precise meanings. Making words work is like carving something functional out of solid material or building a precisely engineered model. It's a technical exercise full of correctness. This is fine as a discipline, but lacks in feeling - an intriguing intellectual exercise, well crafted but lacking. I had no idea of how to develop words and language into the flowing feeling thing I observed in other people. For years I did not know I could do this, the possibility had never been shown to me. Again, that is something I do in my mentoring work. I show autistic people how they can use language with fun, love and the possibilities that go with it.

Even at my engagement party (many years later), my darling wife-to-be, Julie, entertained as well as she could, but I felt exhausted and went to hang out by the wall at the front of the house. Julie came with me, enjoying the quiet. Later we were called back to see family friends and guests in the back garden, where I was asked to make a speech. My response... complete silence. I became frozen to the spot. I had not mentally prepared for this as I did not expect it. I had nothing to use from my vast word database to say how deeply I loved the beautiful young woman, agreeing to be by my side until death do us part. I articulated nothing. I just wanted to die or be swallowed up by the ground.

Faces turned to me. They became still, expecting something from me, and I knew they would be upset if I did not address them, but I was helpless. Public speaking was not something I did in everyday life - all I had ever heard was conversations. There was no model from anything else in my head for this sort of speaking. So I removed myself from the scene with overwhelming feelings of shame. Only with time can I see that it was not my shame to bear. Julie simply slipped her hand in mine and held it tightly, accepting me for who I was, not what the world wanted to see. I hid from family and friends, feeling the weight of judgement upon me as Julie's love fell around me like warm summer rain. Thank you my angel. I adore you more every day and don't tell you enough.

It's not down to persistence, by the way, that I have survived. I put myself up for things and maintain an open life, ready to action whatever happens. That's how I have made connections and got myself into employment - a bit like driving along a road in fog... no overview but prepared to turn off when the next road appears. This happened when I trained to be a Methodist Preacher. I felt a calling to lead people in, encourage and help them understand their faith. In my autistic fashion I appeared at my local church one day saying I was called to do this and ready, because I was.

I remember being asked which preacher I would like to train with, and had no idea, as I don't remember faces well, so couldn't make an informed choice. I had no name to quote either, but I indicated who the person was and that turned out to be the best thing to do. The preacher was called Vic. He was very experienced, passionate and methodical. Just right to train an exceptionally detail-focused autistic person. We got on well.

My next piece of luck came when Vic's wife Marjorie came to a service - I didn't know it but she had recently retired from a teaching career at a London stage school. Marjorie made an appraisal of my speaking form and told me how I was doing. I loved that, it was incredibly useful information. She said I spoke in a monotone voice and needed to slow down a bit, showing me how to inject intonation and styles of speaking. She even offered to train me which made me very pleased – someone bothering to help!

We met weekly for voice exercises, understanding theories of approaching speech, breathing exercises to overcome panic and projection of sound. I saw how to behave and was actually allowed a freedom to 'act' in front of people! This was mind-blowing stuff - how to lead an activity, how to cope and deal with mistakes (without anyone else knowing). After a few months I was voice trained. I could throw my voice, add emotion, ad lib, verbally prepare and practise speaking. It was a revelation and I am very grateful to the time Marjorie spent with me. If only I had been armed with these skills from a younger age, I would have been able to make friends. Naturally, I include this gentle help to all my clients today – old or young. You are never too late to learn!

If you have seen the film *The Kings Speech* you will have seen a story in which Lionel Logue teaches King George VI how to speak. I was trained in exactly the same way, with the same effect. Having a reliable voice is a wonderful thing. It gives you freedom of expression.

Twenty years later I have a well-tuned public voice that's a joy to use. To speak publicly involves using the whole of the body in the best way, including diaphragm breathing, holding the head right, using sinuses, tongue and face to project a versatile, clear human voice. It's something I put my soul into and practice lots (far more than would be apparent when I am speaking). The aim is to appear quite natural, while actually working at a high level of professional competence. This is a skill actors have - they can bring characters alive and the whole thing looks organic and natural complete with emotion - everything woven together to make the character live.

Entrance is of first importance and Marjorie showed me how to step up in front of people. She showed me that their first impression of me and my competence is formed right there and then. That first fraction of a second sets the whole presentation up. One cannot wholly retrieve things if the entrance is not right. Marjorie said the entrance is the point at which the performance peaks. It must be spot on or what follows cannot be as good as it could or should be. A fraction of a second, right at the start, to get everything right. No pressure then... I recognise this trained skill in speakers now and respect what they do. They are so professional in appearing not to be using any skill - and that's what I strive for in my speaking work.

When I am speaking professionally, people are paying good money to hear me – often shocked at an autistic person seeming 'normal'. That's why I talk – more autistic people need to be heard. Autistic novels need to be written by autistics, not non-autistics. Autism-centred plays need to be played by autistic actors, not 'normal' people. My audience deserves value for money and is captivated by my insight into an autistic mind, spoken straight from an autistic mouth. Marjorie helped me no end with my confidence in doing this. She said that the audience are expecting something good, and since the person at the front is supposedly going to deliver something good to the audience, I had not only their permission, but also their willingness, to give me the time and space to perform. They would wait and want the best.

That information is good for calming nerves when out in public. I step up to the mark, fulfil and exceed the audience's expectations. They always remark afterwards about my not using notes or a PowerPoint presentation. Too right I don't use notes, I have rehearsed properly! Any impression I give of being relaxed, with everything flowing naturally, is wholly down to Marjorie's training practice and preparation. And as for PowerPoint - I have a question... do you ever see an actor using PowerPoint, or a script, when they are performing?

I sometimes use computers to help when words are needed physically. Yesterday, I wrote over two thousand words for this book and also read a few emails. I spoke a handful of words to people on the telephone, but writing was the hardest way to use words and I was exhausted by the end of the day. The finished manuscript for this book is over ninety thousand words that needed editing, shaping, and proofing. You needed to know this as a normal person reading autistic work.

There is a letter for me in the post today. It will remain unread for a day or two as I work up to reading it - getting my head in the right place to become tuned for its content. Emails continually eat at my word capacity - even to see if it can be deleted, I must read words. Luckily, my PR agent is a Myers Briggs INFJ type individual who operates with minimal communications - especially for me, ensuring she gets straight to the point (thank you Annie Penn, I am so glad we met). But there is very little respite from words for me, and my capacity to use them gets stretched thin until I become very tired - an uncomfortable, messed up brain 'washed-out' sort of tired.

Spoken words get me through life but I use a certain amount before needing to stop and retreat somewhere silent to re-group myself. There is no need to tie up my vision with seeing and decoding letters to make up words. When I read, I have to scan every word in detail and think about it to be sure I have the right word. Letters are tiring, as are written words. They contain no shape until read and processed into a vision. On the other hand, I love Chinese and Japanese calligraphy for the expressive brush strokes, textures, different depths of ink and beautifully crafted, instantly visual written language via pictogram structure.

The last two paragraphs took so much out of my brain that I have needed a two-hour break before coming back to the computer. They took one and a half hours to write. This rate of writing is typical, and how many hours do you think I have put into this book? While having a break I lay down to stare at the ceiling in a quiet place, going through meditative techniques and shutting my brain chatter off. I reckon I'm good for another hour of writing.

To keep things in order and give me visual interest I open up my web browser and search for visuals to re-tune senses using Flickr - a photo sharing website. I hold lots of visuals there, including my own photo stream (Richard Maguire cycle.nut66) and look up things that hold my concentration. At the moment I am looking for images made using a Leica Summitar 50mm f2 lens. I like the finesse and 3D quality of images made using this lens. I do not have one and intend to buy one with a Leica screw mount body to use it on. I use this as motivation as well - if this book makes enough money I want to buy a Leica Summitar and camera body, as well as help non-autistic people live alongside and work with autistic individuals – that's my goal. I'm a simple soul.

Now for a quick jumping off point - like any human, autistic people need motivation. For us, this motivation will come from our specific and passionate interests. For me, a Leica camera and lens works as my obsessive passion; for another autistic person something else will do as well. I could also be motivated by discussing the *Lord of the Rings* books. (Not the films! Don't forget autistic people are singular in interests and I will not move from the books to the films in a conversation, because they are two vastly different subjects.) Mainly our motivation comes from being passionate about what we do and wanting to make a perfect job of it. We are not bothered about things being hard, we will work though that - our lives are hard and need to be worked through every day with meticulous detail and point-to-point planning. We do not do generalisations, we do many details instead (and that's hard).

Being Out Under The Sky

Here is where I find a sense of freedom for my mind and for my soul.

Out under the sky, the pressures that close in on me - people expecting certain responses, placing expectations that I can only fulfil in part, being social, showing empathy, cooperation through 'normal' (noisy and complex neuro typical) means are lifted for an hour of freedom.

The pressure of 'acting' normal to operate in society causes feelings of anxiety - rooms close in on me, artificial light hurts more than usual, the air seems thicker and breathing is laboured, as if I cannot take in the oxygen I need. I am suffocating.

There is also a further closing in. It attacks me constantly... prickle of bits, things, clutter, shapes, more bits, carpet patterns, pictures, furniture design, papers, cups, stale air, chatter, chatter, chatter, chatter, chatter, chatter, chatter, chatter, chatter, prickle, spike, prickle, suffocating movement, restlessness, noise of clothes rustling, fingers moving, shoes moving, breathing, prickle, spike, yellow tungsten light, lack of visual contrast, too much to see, a queasy colour balance, noise, people's social prickle, chatter, chatter, chatter, movement, nudging. I am in a swirling, Brownian motion of people, but worse because the Brownian motion I feel is sentient, directed, emotional.

People expect responses from me and express dissatisfaction at my poorly formed or absent responses. Faces and people surround me in a clatter and swirl showing rejection, irritation, criticism, more noise and swirl. I feel giddy, sick, in pain, literally and it lasts for ages. I'm panicking inside but hold a straight face, going red, itches hurt, social prickle stings from a glance of confusion. I notice everything going on, all conversations simultaneously, all crockery and glasses chinking, all movement, the noise of people breathing.

Still I am expected to socialise and respond with competence, displaying all sorts of chatter and bonding behaviours. I perceive so much that I do not know when someone is addressing me, and if I do I use all my remaining cognitive abilities trying to understand what they are saying, I am delirious from a place of noise, prickle, chatter, chatter, chatter, chatter, chatter, chatter, clinking, rustling, lights, unnatural colours, low contrast, swirling movement, expectations of me, conversation from me, neuro typical amounts of emotion around me, expected from me. Overloaded, unable to have relationship with anyone, I want relationship, I'm isolated, in pain, and I'm in hell.

What I wrote in the previous paragraph descended into a huge intense and poorly formed sentence. Did you skim it? Did you jump forwards out of it? Was it comprehensible? Did it irritate you by being bad grammar? What was the point? People don't concentrate for that long on something so intense, muddled and poorly structured. Being autistic is like living in this sort of intensity all the time. We go quiet, have meltdowns, avoid social situations, and stand in the corner holding a drink, eyes down, faces detached and brains in overload - in pain.

Being out under the sky, blue, white or grey above, green or brown below, being in the world of nature moving, living all around. The sweet sounds of life, wind, water, birdsong, all music – none of it wants to claim me or thinks it has a claim on me. I feel life everywhere. I notice things neuro typical people overlook. The noise of socialising and chatter masks all this. Out here my hypersensitive soul has rest. None of nature wants me and I fit in. Life goes on... sweet, just right, pure life, sounds (no noise).

Above is the infinity of space, not a ceiling with its horrid yellow strobe light. Wind moves the clouds, lovely patterns and light driven with power. Be still long enough and wait for wild animals to appear.

I photograph in all this. Taken only in photographs, I sit lightly and 'autistically' in this. I do not claim anything. I live in and with it. Being on the cliffs at Llantwit Major while the sun sets over the Bristol Channel. Light appearing over north Devon, watching the sea moving its ships on the incoming tide and a surfer. Here is peace.

'Nothing compares to the simple pleasure of riding a bike.' – John F. Kennedy. Yes, he was right. Riding a bike alone or in company. There is happiness and peace to be found riding a bike. I ride alone lots to experience the motion, feel and effort. All this combines to bring me to a peace I do not find elsewhere. I have a simple single speed bike that moves when I pedal and that's it - pure cycling, silent, free and happy. The bike is built in custom colours, a white frame, blue wheels, and green tyres. Sweet, comfortable colours. I see the front wheel spinning and feel fine. My body fizzing with health, legs spinning, deep breaths taken holding my head up in the countryside.

Hedgerows blur, the horizon reels in, the road curves, moving under the sky. Swooping round corners, whizzing down hills and fizzing fast up them puts the world in tune. Tiredness lifts to make room for being happy. My senses integrate and my mind clears.

I ride in company too. I ride sharing cycling, talking, moving. Cycling together with new and old clients over mentoring sessions means I can get to talk to people that have similar interests as me; I can identify with them and try to make friendships – let them begin to feel connected to break the ice. In the autistic life, pure socialising is hard. So hard that communications and friendships are not possible in most social situations. We do much better when we share an activity, an interest with a form and purpose. Through this we can have a way in to other people's lives and share our own - feeling happier and more human.

For any parents of an autistic child and those that are autistic people-reading, find other people who share your passionate interests. They will gather to share these in clubs or less formally. In these gatherings you can relate, communicate and have friends. The activities provide a route in, shared language and communication. Your interest is an effective way of relaxing enough to cope with a social situation. The drive to do and share your passionate interest gives energy, which can be enough to overcome an internal angst.

In my lowest times in my teens and early 20s, cycling gave just enough hope, exercise, and pain relief to keep me going. I owe a large part of my life to cycling and the people I have met that let me discuss technicalities of bike building. It was my lifeline in my darkest times. I mentor autistic people today and they too find life, love and hope in their passionate interests. Very often we find other autistic people in our interests; this helps, as the social pressure with these people is less, so we succeed more in finding this style of friend.

Like the opening sentence of this chapter, social chat is incomprehensible and painful, but when I am with other cyclists, we chat less and talk more about cycling. Cycling is a subject and that is helpful. We are specific thinkers and it's much easier to start and maintain a conversation on a specific subject. For instance, I often start with a question about cycling and let my client discuss their interest. It's much easier this way. The conversation that follows is normally on subject, less fragmented and easier to process. Even if your audio processing overloads and you miss bits, there is still a better chance of coming back in on the conversation as you will have pre-existing words and knowledge, so getting back in can be done successfully.

Have a listen to 'The Fool on the Hill' by the Beatles. That's me. People have told me I am just a fool in many ways. When they say this, there is pain. For a while I am blinded by the pain. I try to work it out, let it subside, like waiting for nettle rash to fade. Hmm, nettle rash, that's like neuro typical social prickle. People say I am just a fool. Should they take time to listen, they can get rather discomfited by what I know. I am the remote observer. In my quiet I see much, I analyse, I report, I don't sugar coat this. Later in life, my insight and analysis has become valued. I don't play politics - I'm autistic. People who are genuine and do not fear the truth value my insight. Those who play games reject me.

Blah Blah Blah

When out with people I go quite blank most of the time. There is too much information to process. I am able to do a passable impression of being in touch and listening, which works as long as no one wants my attention directly. I am either too overloaded to decode their words and non-verbal communication, or I just don't hear them in all the unfiltered noise and visual stimulation going on all over the place. People's words sound like shattering glass to me - no words are processed, I just perceive tinkling and rumbling sounds.

I will try a stock phrase, or a sentence based on what I think they may be saying, or what I think the situation requires. I often get this wrong, I am constantly stressed at the thought that someone may want to speak to me. What will I do and say? I do like these people and I know they interpret my lack of attention and appropriate language as being unfriendly or ignorant. I just don't behave the way they expect and so I don't make the friendships and connections I want to make. I dislike social situations, but I like the people - so social it has to be if I am to meet people. I will often dip out of a social gathering as I just don't have the strength to cope. I feel sad, though, as I do really like people and want to make friends. This is common in the autistic life.

Out of a crowd, I may hear my wife or someone who knows me say 'wake up', 'stop daydreaming' or 'you're in a world of your own'. My wife says that sometimes I just ignore people or walk away from them and it's perceived as rude. What happens from my perspective is that I just did not recognise them as nearby enough for interaction and that they wanted inclusion. I will not even identify their voices or any gestures they make to me.

One-to-one and conversations can be fine, but add one person and I struggle to manage (if the words do not come too fast). Add one more person into the mix and my processing is overloaded. I try to tune in to one person at a time and piece together an understanding of the conversation. That works for a while until white noise, intonation speech, movement, facial expressions and pressure to interact become too much. Shutdown or silent meltdown ensues. That means I find coping mechanisms internally, and acting normal is enforced until escape situations present an opportunity to flee.

In a group of people, I am not processing anything more than their positions alongside overall noise level and physical placement in the immediate environment. I try to appear normal and say stuff to join in, but it's hard when I am not following the conversation. I look at people and check my mental database to see if I can recognise when to speak and what I could say. I am simply reading minimal placement and noise level information.

It's strange, this not perceiving people or things when I am overloaded. The feeling is like being a little drunk. The room does not seem real. People move and make sounds, but I cannot process this and decode. I see things clearly, yet don't if that makes any sense. I see an ear, some hair, a clothing seam, a hand etc. One movement, however, that does not add up to reading the whole scene is confusing when trying to piece together a 'whole'. There is too much in my vision everywhere I look. It all hurts; the room is not stable; I cannot judge distance very well, and I am unaware of time.

The whole experience feels awful. I want to be ill and I feel like I am going to fall over - my balance is struggling with the overload. I normally lean to the right and veer to the right. If walking when this happens, I try to be near a wall for comfort and to steady myself.

Then there is sound, all pervasive, I cannot turn it off or look away. It hurts, it stings, it screeches and it throbs. Pain, pain, pain. Out of this, someone will be saying something to me that I dimly sense, like a sound coming up a long tube, distorted and whooshing on the air. Ouch, it hurts too, but there is more pain here. The person wants me to understand what they have said and wants me to respond in a friendly way, but I am doing my best to hide the pain. The pain increases because I cannot do this naturally and I know they will be disappointed, which can give them a poor opinion of me. Pain grows deep inside; I feel ill and want to leave, but usually I am frozen to the spot like a rabbit in the headlights.

It hurts writing this for you to read and process in your own way. I feel nauseous and am putting a lot of effort into explaining it all so that people who read this will know and understand something of the autistic world. We simply do not do rude, arrogant or ignorant.

The trouble is that people interpret our behaviour based on normal social rules and understandings. This, I believe, is at the root of why autism is so disabling for those of us who are autistic. We go through life in a constant round of social faux pas, misunderstandings and trouble. This irks and disturbs people around us, causing them to dislike our company and to put distance between them and us. We just cannot be understood by normal social rules, but this is tried every day by people who interact with us. We know this and put a lot of effort into interacting, hoping things will go well with other people.

So back to 'Blah Blah Blah'. This is as close as I can describe my perception of people's communication to me in crowded environments. Crowded can be two or more people, depending on the circumstance. This evening I was put into overload by just two people. I was tired and just could not decode their communication, let alone process it, yet they wanted a normal response from me at each interaction. I was unable to supply the response they wanted. I perceived their dissatisfaction with me. They had become stereo 'Blah Blah Blah'. Each sentence and movement from them stung me and wrung at my soul. They are people I know and love well, and if they would be still, still enough for an autistic person, which is very still indeed, I would be so happy in their company.

If you can read to the end of this chapter you will have a great hunger to understand the actions of an autistic person and a clear sense of what they are experiencing in a social setting. What follows is what I endure in social gatherings – wherever they are. I have no means to filter sensory inputs - they all come along at the same volume and brightness. I am hypersensitive on all my senses - everything is very loud to me at all time and in all places.

Written below is what I hear when lots of people are around me. Also imagine the echo in a room and the noises of feet shuffling, clothes rustling, people scratching, crockery clinking and more. Everything is loud to me; there is no quiet. I can hear every sound someone makes. One of the loudest sounds to me is the noise of their clothes as they move. Their voice is way back underneath an overlay of sounds. 'Blah blah blah' is the fumbling soft sounds of speech, the creak and crackle is hard and high pitched, similar to the sound of breaking glass.

I hear… Blah blah blah blah blah blah blah plink critch creak plack blal balah balah rhubarb rhubarb rhubarb pock wahah weeh murble lackblah blah blah blah blah blah blah blah blah woop ablah ablah balah blah balah ablaha blah ablib plik whahahah wahaha ablah ab;lah ablah weeeeng plack scritch we he BLAH ABHAL BLAH wick pack scree pip blah blah blah blah blah blah blah blah blah blah ablah blah blah blah blah blah blah ablah wip scrik weih wieh scree wek weeh plick mak blah blah blah ablla ablah ablah blah blah ablah blah ablah balah ablah woops crick week wik wah wik wik wehehehehhee Blah ablah blah blah blah cak plik cak cak plik weeh weeh weeh wah wah Blah blah wik wik scree wahahaha wik screes wahhha scree plik plick waha blah blah blah blah blah blah blah blah blah blah blah blah blah blah blah blah blah blah blah blah blah blah blah blah blah blah blah blah blah blah blah blah blah blah blah blah blah blah

blah blah blah blah blah blah blah blah blah blah blah blah blah
blah blah blah blah blah blah blah blah blah blah blah blah blah
blah blah blah blah blah blah blah blah blah blah blah blah blah
blah blah blah blah blah blah blah blah blah Blah blah blah blah
blah blah blah plink critch creak plack blal balah balah rhubarb
rhubarb rhubarb pock wahah weeh murble lackblah blah blah
blah blah blah blah blah blah woop ablah ablah balah blah balah
ablaha blah ablib plik whahahah wahaha ablah ab;lah ablah
weeeeng plack scritch we he BLAH ABHAL BLAH wick pack scree
pip blah blah blah blah blah blah blah blah blah blah blah ablah
blah blah blah blah blah blah ablah wip scrik weih wieh scree wek
weeh plick mak blah blah blah blah ablla ablah ablah blah blah
ablah blah ablah balah ablah Blah blah blah blah blah blah blah
plink critch creak plack blal balah balah footall rhubarb rhubarb
rhubarb pock wahah weeh murble lackblah blah blah blah blah
blah blah blah blah woop ablah ablah balah blah balah ablaha
blah ablib plik whahahah wahaha ablah ab;lah ablah weeeeng
plack scritch we he BLAH ABHAL BLAH wick pack scree pip blah
blah blah blah blah blah blah blah blah blah blah ablah blah blah
blah blah blah blah ablah wip scrik weih wieh scree wek weeh
plick mak blah blah blah blah ablla ablah ablah blah blah ablah
blah ablah balah ablah Blah blah blah blah blah blah blah plink
critch creak plack blal balah balah rhubarb rhubarb rhubarb pock
wahah weeh murble lackblah blah blah blah blah blah blah blah
blah woop ablah ablah balah blah balah ablaha blah ablib plik
whahahah wahaha ablah ab;lah ablah weeeeng plack scritch we
he BLAH ABHAL BLAH wick pack scree pip blah blah blah blah blah
blah blah blah blah blah ablah blah blah blah blah blah blah blah
ablah wip scrik weih wieh scree wek weeh plick mak blah blah
blah blah ablla ablah ablah blah blah ablah blah ablah balah ablah
stop daydreaming Blah blah blah blah blah blah blah plink critch
creak plack blal balah balah rhubarb rhubarb rhubarb pock wahah
weeh murble lackblah blah blah blah blah blah blah blah
woop ablah ablah balah blah balah ablaha blah ablib plik
whahahah wahaha ablah ab;lah ablah weeeeng plack scritch we
he BLAH ABHAL BLAH wick pack scree pip blah blah blah blah blah

blah blah blah blah blah blah ablah blah blah blah blah blah blah
ablah wip scrik weih wieh scree wek weeh plick mak blah blah
blah blah ablla ablah ablah blah blah ablah blah ablah balah ablah
ablaha blah ablib plik whahahah wahaha ablah ab;lah ablah
weeeeng plack scritch we he BLAH ABHAL BLAH wick pack scree
pip blah blah blah blah blah blah blah blah blah blah blah ablah
blah blah blah blah blah blah ablah wip scrik weih wieh scree wek
weeh plick mak blah blah blah blah ablla ablah ablah blah blah
ablah blah ablah balah ablah ablaha blah ablib plik whahahah
wahaha ablah ab;lah ablah weeeeng plack scritch we he BLAH
ABHAL BLAH wick pack scree pip blah blah blah blah blah blah
blah blah blah blah blah ablah blah blah blah blah blah blah ablah
blah blah plink critch creak plack blal balah balah rhubarb rhubarb
rhubarb pock wahah weeh murble lackblah blah blah blah blah
blah blah blah blah woop ablah ablah balah blah balah ablaha
blah ablib plik whahahah wahaha ablah ab;lah ablah weeeeng
plack scritch we he BLAH ABHAL BLAH wick pack scree pip blah
blah blah blah blah blah blah blah blah blah ablah blah blah
blah blah blah blah ablah wip scrik weih wieh scree wek weeh
plick mak blah blah blah blah ablla ablah ablah blah blah ablah
blah ablah balah ablah woops crick week wik wah wik wik
wehehehehhee Blah ablah blah blah Blah blah blah blah blah blah
blah plink critch creak plack blal balah balah rhubarb rhubarb
come on rhubarb pock wahah weeh murble lackblah blah blah
blah blah blah blah blah woop ablah ablah balah blah balah
ablaha blah ablib plik whahahah wahaha ablah ab;lah ablah
weeeeng plack scritch we he BLAH ABHAL BLAH wick pack scree
pip blah blah blah blah blah blah blah blah blah blah blah ablah
blah blah blah blah blah blah ablah wip scrik weih wieh scree wek
weeh plick mak blah blah blah blah ablla ablah ablah blah blah
ablah blah ablah balah ablah woops crick week wik wah wik wik
wehehehehhee Blah ablah blah blah don't you think? Blah blah
blah blah blah blah blah plink critch creak plack blal balah balah
rhubarb rhubarb rhubarb pock wahah weeh murble lackblah blah
blah blah blah blah blah blah blah woop ablah ablah balah blah
balah ablaha blah ablib plik whahahah wahaha ablah ab;lah ablah

weeeeng plack scritch we he BLAH ABHAL BLAH wick pack scree
pip blah blah blah blah blah blah blah blah blah blah blah ablah
blah blah blah blah blah blah ablah wip scrik weih wieh scree wek
weeh plick mak blah blah blah blah ablla ablah ablah blah blah
ablah blah ablah balah ablah woops crick week wik wah wik wik
wehehehehhee Blah ablah blah blah blah blah blah blah blah blah
plink critch creak plack blal balah balah rhubarb rhubarb rhubarb
pock wahah weeh murble lackblah blah blah blah rhubarb pock
wahah weeh murble lackblah blah blah blah blah blah blah blah
blah woop ablah ablah balah blah balah ablaha blah ablib plik
whahahah wahaha ablah ab;lah ablah weeeeng plack scritch we
he BLAH ABHAL BLAH wick pack scree pip blah blah blah blah blah
blah blah blah blah blah ablah blah blah blah blah blah blah
ablah wip scrik weih wieh scree wek weeh plick mak blah blah
blah blah ablla ablah ablah blah blah ablah blah ablah balah ablah
woops crick week wik wah wik wik wehehehehhee Blah ablah
blah blah blah cak plik cak cak plik weeh weeh weeh wah wah
Blah blah blah blah blah blah blah blah blah blah blah blah blah
blah blah blah blah blah blah blah blah blah blah blah blah blah
blah blah blah blah blah blah blah blah blah blah blah blah blah
blah blah blah blah blah blah blah blah blah blah blah blah blah
blah blah blah blah blah blah blah blah blah blah blah blah blah
blah wik wik scree wahahaha wik screes wahhha scree plik plick
waha blah blah blah blah blah blah blah blah blah blah blah blah
blah blah blah blah blah blah blah blah blah blah blah blah blah
blah blah blah blah blah blah blah blah blah blah blah blah blah
blah blah blah blah blah blah blah blah blah blah blah blah blah
blah blah blah blah blah blah blah blah blah blah blah blah blah
blah blah blah blah blah blah blah blah blah blah blah blah blah
blah Blah blah blah blah blah blah blah plink critch creak plack blal
balah balah rhubarb rhubarb rhubarb pock wahah weeh murble
lackblah blah blah blah blah blah blah blah blah woop ablah ablah
balah blah balah ablaha blah ablib plik whahahah wahaha ablah
ab;lah ablah weeeeng plack scritch we he BLAH ABHAL BLAH wick
pack scree pip blah blah blah blah blah blah blah blah blah blah
blah ablah blah blah blah blah blah blah ablah wip scrik weih wieh

scree wek weeh plick mak blah blah blah blah ablla ablah ablah
blah blah ablah blah ablah balah ablah Blah blah blah blah blah
blah blah plink critch creak plack blal balah balah footall rhubarb
rhubarb rhubarb pock wahah weeh murble lackblah blah blah
blah blah blah blah blah blah woop ablah ablah balah blah balah
ablaha blah ablib plik whahahah wahaha ablah ab;lah ablah
weeeeng plack scritch we he BLAH ABHAL BLAH wick pack scree
pip blah blah blah blah blah blah blah blah blah blah blah ablah
blah blah blah blah blah blah ablah wip scrik weih wieh scree wek
weeh plick mak blah blah blah blah ablla ablah ablah blah blah
ablah blah ablah balah ablah Blah blah blah blah blah blah blah
plink critch creak plack blal balah balah rhubarb rhubarb rhubarb
pock wahah weeh murble lackblah blah blah blah blah blah blah
blah blah woop ablah ablah balah blah blah blah blah blah blah
woop wehehehehhee and so on, and so on, until the torture ends
when I can get out of the situation.

The above text really is as much sense as I can make of social
gatherings. They are as tedious as this writing, punctuated with
out-of-context words that people assume I am understanding, and
can fit in to the social whole.

And, yes, I do pick up criticisms of me. They hurt, but I cannot be
too bothered about them right there 'in the moment', as it means
extra hurt to process. I do my embarrassment and hurting later on
- hours, weeks, months and years later. I really do like the people,
but cannot communicate or handle social gatherings. This has
been the case all my life. Please imagine the above alongside
visual overload and a disturbed vestibular system.

I am not rude, aloof, ignorant or unfriendly. I am in pain. It's just
that most people will not recognise the pain I suffer and put my
lack of interaction down to some sort of rudeness.

Captain Pugwash And How I Learned To Read

I do not learn words phonetically. I learn the shape and the sound that goes with the shape. I suppose I read written text in the way ancient Egyptians read hieroglyphs: the shape stands for a word. When learning to read and write at school, I remember looking over at other children's work, seeing the word shape they put in their exercise book and listening for the word sound. Then I would copy the shape and attach the sound to it.

That was how I got round being expected to learn phonetics. I recall cringing when the letters for the day were written on the blackboard. Then, later in the day, the teacher would use the letter of the day with other letters to make sounds and syllables. I learned little from this and tried not to get noticed in this part of the lesson, but it resulted in my being noticed and subsequent rebuking for not knowing what to say or do. That would also lead on into the playground as fuel for more bullying.

I had a double reason not to interact in these sound-forming parts of the lessons. I tried to lay low until the end when the teacher would give us the words. I simply copied the words and attached the sound. Bingo: several new words in one! If I survived the lesson, it was a success and I would not be told off for being lazy or not paying attention. I wished the teacher would just write up the word and tell us what it was - that would save lots of time with all the muddle and unclear stuff going on in between.

So much of school was about lying low like this, trying to be ignored until I could get exactly what the lessons were about. I am still like this today, I would rather be told something then go away and figure its details out with research and related subjects. In common with a lot of autistic people, I do not get on very well with classroom-based interactive learning and group work. I am okay on my own though, and a lot of us would rather be taught in ways that are not considered good classroom practice.

Interactive learning and group work overloads autistic children through our trying to get to grips with all the movement, social negotiations, people, chatter and processing the activities. After dealing with this amount of sensory overload, a lot of us haven't got any spare brain capacity left to learn the subject - we are burned out trying to cope with the social life of the classroom.

Multi-sensory and kinaesthetic learning is good for some, as is quiet lone study with some direction from a teacher. But we would rather do this away from distraction, language, movement, people, and noise and sensory overload. Most autistic children are good at experimenting and exploring subjects and we prefer this approach. Put us in a noisy, crowded environment and that's it, game over, as we are not learning we are surviving.

School was like this for me. It was a place to be endured, a place of confusion and pain. I was expected to learn new things. People knew I was intelligent and got angry with me when I failed to show evidence of learning. The few old school reports I have are painful reading. There was the occasional highlight such as art, history and geology, but the rest was horrid wrongful judgement of a bright boy trapped by pain.

Let's get back to learning phonetics. I was not going anywhere with this system and became a class joke, relegated to looking at lower level reading books than the rest. They took an age to read and I had no idea what I was to learn from each book. Besides, I wasn't interested in knowing that Janet and John went to the shops to buy mother a loaf of bread. I would be far more interested in all the background information, like how the bread was made, what were the makes of the cars in the street and so on. The pictures were good and did get my attention. I wished I was like John; he seemed to get on well in life. But I still did not get the text or recognise any new words, and grammar. I have just had to look up 'grammar' for this manuscript and apply the principles – please forgive me for being inadequate if at all incorrect. My point is to convey the sightless methodology of educational institutions balanced against a frightened autistic child who wants to learn in order to become a useful part of society.

I can use language through practice, observation, feedback and repetition, but I have never been able to learn the rules of English grammar in themselves. I do not know what a verb is, nor a pronoun, nor any of those kinds of things. I have been taught, but I just don't get a cognitive handle on them. In fact, I don't learn rules very well. I can get to grips with reality but not the underlying rules – this applies in life or in team games. I build up a matrix of facts I can refer to so I appear to know the rules.

I remember my parents talking to each other about my lack of progress at school. Some of it was put down to laziness. I didn't do lazy, but what I did do was depressed and hours of lost hope in the classroom. I did not know the rules or how to do things at school. I was only vaguely aware of the purpose of school. I was just sent there and it was horrid. I knew words like class and lesson, but I was only distantly connected with what they were about, or what I should do or gain from them. I was lost, and outside of things I got bullied - that didn't help me learn. Most of the time I just hated going anywhere near school and had no idea how I would benefit from it. Just to see the school, go near it, or to talk about it at home, scared me. I learned lots as a young child but very little of it at school.

My strategy a lot of the time at school was to isolate myself from within. To go to a little place deep inside only I knew about, not connected with the dreadful physical or mental reality in school. Comments were made about how quiet and well-behaved I was. Quiet was good, it meant peace and retreat. Not learn, just live there.

A top tip is to check what kind of quiet a child is living in. There are two sorts. One is a peaceful quiet. The other that I and many autistic children display is a *dead quiet*. They differ in feel - the former is soft, with a discernible peace. The child can slip in and out of it being able to communicate and engage with a seamless air. The latter is deep, has an air of disconnection, like staring into a deep black pool without reflection or acknowledgement that you are there and looking in.

There is also no ease when coming out of the quiet. The child will display a jerky, scratchy route, hesitant, back into life outside the quiet. Transition is from a small sad place of safety back into the world that carries the fear of death, shows the fear of horrors the world holds – waiting for you to return. Be aware also that this applies to frightened, unhappy adults as well, be they autistic or suffering for any other reason.

The concern over my inability to read and write was getting stronger at home. I too got worried, as I knew reading and writing were important skills. I knew I had to master them if I wanted to go to university, study interesting things and do an interesting job. I was scared at the prospect of leaving school with very little and getting into dead end jobs that would not use my intellect. That was the situation I found myself in as school ended.

A house not far away from ours was number 007, which I thought was cool. In it lived a teacher called Hillary. I was aware that my mum was talking to her about my lack of progress with reading and writing, and recall Hillary talking to me one day about this (my parents were there too). Now I know she had been asked to see if she could help, but as a young autistic boy I had no idea what was going on, and could not guess as no one told me. I did not make these connections.

One day before school, my mum told me to go to see Hillary on my way home. I still had no idea why and it brings me to make a request - if you are a parent or teacher of an autistic child, please do not assume the child has a framework for knowing what is going on. Their perceptions of life and knowledge are very fragmented and they will not have developed much ability to see these connections. Please just tell them, as it will help more than you could know, even if it is blindingly obvious and simple - please tell them anyway. These things are a mystery to the child who is not making the connections in their fragmented world.

I went to see Hillary after school and was busting for the toilet, but I had not realised I could ask to go. I did not use the toilets much at school because of bullies. So many times, I went to these extra lessons just bursting to go, but did not know I could ask or even how to ask. I lost a lot of concentration because of this. An autistic kid won't know to ask even about the simplest things, and may be holding onto intolerable situations and not know how to say, or that they can say, or that words can be used to communicate. They are normally suffering in silence - this goes on into adulthood too. This can so often be another reason the autistic child is failing to thrive and learn.

Hillary's dining room was a lot better than a classroom full of noisy children (although I had not yet figured out that I was sent there to learn). I did not make a connection between this and other ways of learning - it was all in a new context to which I could not transfer other knowledge. I was interested in her reading books as I believed reading books were basic Janet and John books. I had no idea that other books were reading books too!

The books Hillary had were a pirate reading book series and Captain Pugwash books. I liked anything about pirates and Captain Pugwash, as a character in a popular children's cartoon series in the early 1970's. He was pompous and incompetent and the rest of his crew were equally incompetent. The only person keeping his ship The Black Pig in order was Tom, the cabin boy. Tom was the only crew member with any sense, but no one would give Tom credit for anything. I identified with Tom. I never got credit for things. I was seen as the junior and less competent partner in any enterprise, just like Tom, but if anyone would ask me I did have lots of answers and insight.

Now here was the key to my learning... the pirate books and Captain Pugwash stories. Do remember that we autistic people have passionate interests in certain things. When educating us, especially as children, please find out what our passion is, and link a lot of learning to it. And, no, it is not an obsession that needs to be discouraged (do that and we will end up lost, without a passion for attaching all kinds of knowledge and skills to).

I got on with Captain Pugwash stories and I started to read. I used to mentally blank out when Hillary was breaking words down into their phonetics and wait until she told me the word, pretending that I had grasped it through phonetics. I was expected to find phonetics easy and useful but I hated it. In the one-to-one style of teaching in a quiet space that made up Hillary's dining room I built sentences and started to read. I learned quickly and am very grateful for that opportunity, I have no idea how or when I would have learned to read otherwise.

College

I hoped a clean start in a new place with new people would work. I checked out a local sixth form and the local college, deciding on college, as there appeared to be fewer organisational expectations of me. I felt nervous and held on to a hope that I could rescue my education and go to university. I still clung to a desire to be an expert in something and find fulfilment mentally as well as an income. I knew I had a creative and interested intellect, but had not yet been able to put anything on paper that came close to my abilities, and I had no idea why.

I started to study for two A-levels – geography and history, because I had an affinity for these subjects. (I really wanted to do Geology but did not have the maths.) I also hoped that the new environment and culture might help me meet people and shake off my reputation as an outsider.

I started off keen and ready to learn. The layout of the place confused me, but I found this useful for being able to approach people. However these openings dried up by the end of the second week. Then I was aware that fellow students were forming relationships and I had not managed this. I had not managed to get beyond initial greetings. Getting into conversation and forming relationships with new people has always been hard; when the conversation turns after the greeting I simply cannot follow it. I felt low and despondent at this point. Was history repeating itself? I had a sinking feeling it was. There had been a change of environment, but no change in me. The same old things that held me back before surfaced again.

I also found studying difficult as I had no template to follow and insufficient organisational skills to get on with it. No amount of folders, pages subject headings and constant internal repetition of subjects and study skills worked. A familiar lack of organisation saw to that. No external structure or environment affected this. I loved my subjects and had plenty of interest in exploring the theory. However, my notes were a mess or completely lacking, and I had no idea how to follow the text books as a study guide in note form. This is one of the main concepts I will show an autistic child when mentoring them today. Skills needed to absorb and recall subject matter from theoretical materials and subsequent lectures.

I was aware that study at college level required me to do research with little guidance - that was fine, as I saw it as an adventure, but for a reason I did not follow a coordinated approach and it became impossible. Unaware I was autistic, I was behind in other areas without the means to seek support. Not that there was any educational support of the kind I needed back then. Nor was any sort of diagnosis possible. I did I know what on earth was wrong with me, I just knew it was not right.

How could I facilitate my brain into engaging my already high IQ and ability to reason with presenting findings and ideas? The situation was desperate - I constantly felt as if I was stuck in quicksand, struggling hard and getting deeper into difficulty. I strived for achievement without success and no clues as to why eventually becoming diagnosed with depression. A diagnosis was some years off. My hope, enthusiasm and confidence waned. I knew I had the few years that these courses lasted to do something, and then it was off out of education and into a dead end job. Into a life of ?????

I knew people who did interesting things for a living, who had degrees. They were my intellectual peers and I knew that they had got into the occupations that they had through study, training and liberating their gifts. I knew that I could do what they were doing, but how? How would a school and college failure persuade anyone that I was worth taking on? Looking back now, I do not think I was able to take anything on back then. I was depressed, socially and developmentally, way behind where I needed to be. I don't think I could have picked up much skill in the workplace and it would have gone the same way as my education had gone.

I was interested to learn decades later that the late teens and early twenties are an especially difficult time for young autistic adults. We are not up to speed in lots of developmental areas. We still have a long way to go, but are expected to be like everyone else at this age, getting on with higher education or getting into work. We are often deeply depressed and have no hope for the future. People around us tend to assume we are lazy and not moving on with life. This was the message I got. This deepened my depression and sense of worthlessness. I just hung on knowing I had two years to go – willing things to get better, but unable to action positive progression. Lots of this was due to my lack of social imagination. I did not know how to interact or influence people.

I went through motions of study; I went to lectures. I dragged my bag that should have had books and notes in around the campus. I went to the refectory, ate on my own, and cycled to and from college on my own. I so wanted to enter the world that other students lived in. I never felt so alone. I used this time as a bit of space between now and the inevitable failure and dead end job.

While at college I used to spend a lot of my time in the pottery studio. I have always been a good 3D thinker and working in clay was a great thing to do. I always had an aptitude for making things. I could do this, so I put in lots of the energy I would have put into study. At least I could do this and I knew my way around a pottery workshop. During the two and a half years I was there I made animal sculptures. I could relate to animals. Then I made a model windmill. Not any model, but one with all the parts in it, all beams and planks, teeth, shafts, stones, chutes and bins. It is a model of a post mill. I made the post and body separately so it would rotate like a real mill. I also made a wind shaft, brake and sails.

The sails had to be made of wood. A far as I could get it, everything worked like a real mill. It weighed a ton and would only just fit in the kiln. I wanted a completed project to prove to myself that I could do something. I wanted something I had made to be admired. The windmill was. It lived on the side in the studio for a month or so. People could scarcely believe something like this could be attempted in ceramics. It had 206 ceramic components, all of which needed to fit together on final assembly, plus the sails. I still have the mill. It is packed in component parts (my house is too small to put it up) and it is stored at my parents' house. It has only been erected twice since college.

The pottery lecturer, Mr Francis, was a hero of mine. He was one of these people who would gently encourage talent out of individuals. He showed me skills that I have used well in the rest of my life - gentle instruction and respect for everyone became my inspiration. Through these dark years he believed in me and helped me to liberate my talents. After the windmill body survived its post-glaze-firing he shared his worry that he didn't think I would pull my project off. He had never seen such a large and complex piece with so many parts, thicknesses and apertures be fired before, and feared it would crack in the kiln.

It survived. Now it may seem strange, but I always knew it would. I have an innate feeling for materials and structures. I knew the clay would hold out, I just knew it, deep in my being. I had handled the clay and had a good measure of its properties so was in no doubt that this carefully designed structure would do the job it had been designed for. I paid special attention to fitting the panels and beams together. I pugged and rolled the clay with special care. I made up my own slips and joined everything with meticulous attention to detail. I knew that any failure would be from lack of preparation or poor method in the build. I had all these covered so I knew it would all be ok. I just knew. And it was.

This success with pottery and making things were the thread that got me through this time in my life. I make, I mend, and I think and create and live. The making I did at college gave me the time and means to think creatively as well. Much of the thinking I did back then is with me now, refined and built on, or completely changed ready for use today.

I tried to learn as well, but the cultural and developmental gaps between me and other students were too big to bridge. I had no comprehension of their lives, communication or means of living. I was the same age and a million years apart in development. I could not communicate in classes. I felt fear and sadness; I was too frightened to absorb the subjects I loved and slid deeper into depression. I stopped learning and attending classes. Getting up each day became harder - the analgesic effects of alcohol became a relief from depression. I recall leaving my bag of notes and essays under some lockers in a corridor. I was too depressed to retrieve them. The bag was taken and my notes scattered on the floor. I had no use for them, no reason to retrieve them.

Field trips let me believe I could get some traction on my subjects through them. A history trip to Exeter University and Finch's Foundry early on gave me renewed interest in my studies. Field trips are kinaesthetic, multi-sensory and offer exploration of the subject outside of a classroom - my favoured ways of learning! Two more trips to Wales - one based near Swansea taking in the Gower Peninsula, where I recall holidays in the 1960's. A trek to Pwlldu Bay to measure beach shingle took me back, so far I was miles away in my mind and soul from the tasks we had to do. But I learned there, out in the Welsh wind and scenery. There was peace enough to engage.

Another geography trip to Llandudno; the Welsh coast, mountains, rivers and woods called my interest into action as I again felt a deep sense of peace there, which contrasted with the widening gap between me and the rest of life. Students I liked stayed distant, as I could not relate to them and their friendships were beyond me. I clung to a faint dream of going to university and growing up in a happy life. At the same time, feeling scared at the distance between me and the life being lived by the students I was with. This was brought into focus by being away from home, living in unpredictable surroundings in the hotel. Depression and pain deadened by alcohol. Dreams left in sorrow. From then on I stopped studying, exhausted and in pain with no idea of a way forward.

I have beautiful photographs from those field trips - there was a real joy in the composition, then as now. I will constantly tell you that if you want to engage an autistic person in conversation, our passionate interests are the way to go. Even in the darkest times there can still be light and engagement through our passions, and it was the case back in my college days, but no one knew, not even me. Life became defined by my lack of progress.

This happens to most of us living with a syndrome – be that autistically born or not. I have been able to help autistic people up from a pit of despair through their passionate interests, and the happiness that results is incredibly rewarding. Happiness and engagement are real keys to life in the autistic world. Please use them and be positive, whatever your connection to autism is. Life comes from this.

In the end, all I had were my passionate interests, photography, cycling and pottery. They kept me alive and were the thread through which I maintained life - proving to myself that I still lived. Over thirty years on, I have not been back to a pottery studio, but still cycle daily and take photographs constantly. In fact, I carry a camera with me at all times – along with my Christian faith. I think the pottery passion came from proving I could do something others doubted would happen.

Sadly, college was where my dreams died and all hope stopped. I remember crying on my way home many times after I knew for sure my dreams of university had died. I had no plans for the future and no idea how I could make a success of my life in ways other than what I knew then - school, university and a well-paid interesting job.

Being autistic, I am a linear thinker and do not perceive alternatives. If no one tells me there are other options and ways round things, I see a full stop. I have taken this lesson into my working life and my situation back then is common in the autistic world. We develop slower than other people and need more creative ways of getting on a result. Today, I help young autistic people learn different paths to find happiness in life. I rekindle hope in them, and fuel them with direction. It is in our own idiosyncratic ways that we discover what works for us.

We do not and cannot follow conventional ways of living – autistics are not wired up for that. Many of us come to grief because people think they are helping us by trying to form us into images of normality and conformity, or what they perceive as normal. As a result we believe we are faulty, get depressed and consider suicide. But we are happy to try ways of connecting and getting on in the rest of life when we are in a good place and know how this will make life better. We can be surprisingly happy and accommodating; this happens when we feel good about who we are. This is most of the work I do. Autism is not a behavioural or medical issue, it's a way of being alive and human.

College ended in 1985. After missing my exams, I knew I was in no state to deal with them and needed a job, so I worked in a DIY store.

Colours

Colours are always together in a beautiful relationship and a living light, something that does my autism and visual sensitivity a lot of good. It's not bright colours as such that overload me, but discordant colours - incomplete light sources like fluorescent lights that overload and hurt. I am happy with a lot of colour. When viewed together, my photographs are very colourful and all the colours sing out in harmony.

Colours are like notes in music that entice me to look for sweet chords and melodies. Beautiful colour combinations dance, intrigue and comfort. Listen to Vaughan Williams *Lark Ascending* for a musical representation of the way I listen to colours.

All my life I have sought and combined colours. I have used toy cars, paints, buttons, lights, cellophane, glass, liquids, flowers (I love arranging flowers, self-taught, looking for colour partnerships in the flowers), mugs in the kitchen cupboard, bowls of fruit, a high street with its shop signs, spring and summer flowers, new green leaves in spring and the deep blue sky.

I see colours as form and life; my camera is often aimed at colours. My photographs have colour chords, colour forms and colour emotions in them. My detail-searching mind sees and follows colour all the time. Sometimes I see colour more than physical form unless the form is brought to life by colours.

I wrestle with black and white photography, it removes colour, and dials out emotion for me, but I love what it does convey by black and white pictures. Yet in life I see colours so vividly, I struggle to see the tones alone. To find the tones I put a coloured filter over the lens so I see one colour only. That way, tones come to life and forms are visible. People photograph so well in black and white that I make the effort, and though black and white pictures resonate with me and I am also able to taste them - synaesthesia. I relate to a colour when it has a taste and a sound. Monochrome has become to me like a subtle savoury taste, similar to mozzarella cheese. With this taste monochrome becomes real.

I seek strong colours in small forms, like jewels, tiny beautiful sweet colours. They taste like boiled sweets. On my desk I have a small propelling pencil with deep red at each end, two cameras with shutter buttons in red, and a red LED light on each. I look into the small red forms and feel sweet energy, while tasting strawberry. I have a camera a Canon AV-1. On the top plate, there is a red A on a round piano-black control dial. At the front there is a tiny, deep red lens for the self-timer light. I look at the two deep reds, feeling happy, having the taste of strawberries in my mouth. I carry this camera as a stim (stimulating) object a lot of the time.

I seek and linger by jewel-like colours, coloured lights. I remember the freezer in the kitchen; I was about three. I loved the coloured lights on the control panel. One day I wanted to explore the lights and carry one with me, so used a kitchen knife to pry one off – bang! An orange flash slammed me into the kitchen cupboards and I found out about being electrocuted. I never expected that, and I remember the burns on my thumb and forefinger. Since then I have been determined to get small coloured, translucent stim objects (avoided the ones connected to mains electricity) such as marbles for their colours.

Whenever I can, I surround myself with blue and green. As a boy I asked my father to paint my bedroom blue and green on alternate walls. Blue and green are the colours of leaves and sky. I relax and fill up with a soft calm, my brain slows and peace can glide in as a result. I taste vanilla when I see these colours. I seek blue and green out in any situation as it helps me to look and avoid visual overload. I have looked long at green fields and blue skies, wanted blue clothes, bought a blue-framed bicycle, blue cars, green files and folders and things for the house. Our current house is pale blue in most rooms, blue carpets with a green one in the lounge.

Orange is hard to look at, and I avoid anything orange. I am writing all this because these things are clues as to the nature of the scotopic sensitivity I, and many autistics, have, seeking blue and green and avoiding orange. I hate artificial light and have even found daylight not quite comfortable. I was middle aged when I went to a specialist optometrist, Michael Blackstone in Beaconsfield (England). We spent time looking into a total colorimeter and the colours that made my vision comfortable were blue and turquoise. All the preference for blue and green and avoidance of orange made sense. I have difficulty processing orange, which my blue and turquoise glasses filter out. My coloured glasses make vision sweet; my ten o'clock headaches stopped; I could read more clearly and daylight was comfortable with the orange light removed.

I am often asked how similar visual processing difficulties can be spotted. There are signs in someone's life that sensory sensitivities and processing issues exist. Is there an attraction to certain sensory inputs and aversion to others? In my life, my liking for blue and green were indicators of my visual processing issues.

I like strong colours in small amounts, marbles, tell-tale lights, LED lights, a deeply coloured car at a distance, flowers in a garden, enamelled objects and camera viewfinder LED lights. On a large scale, anything other than blue, green or brown is too much.

Colour combinations are important too. At Christmas, the decorations are too much, wrapping paper has too many bits of colour, often with a background of red and green, too much rich colour all unsorted in an uncomfortable mixed up mess of colour, bright stuff and overload. At Christmas, my processing of colour begins to break down. Decorated rooms become unbearable, confusing, and headaches are ever present. It is hard to perceive people in this colour overload.

People want to be together in rooms and chatter in a jolly way. Their voices become like shattering glass, and colours hurt in all directions. I do not know where to look. I feel pain and become disorientated when red and green are next to each other. Horrid tastes come along with pain in my forehead and visual confusion. This colour combination is predominant at Christmas - for a month every year I must contend with red/green combination pain. Then people insist on me being jolly and festive, yet Christmas hurts every year.

On the other hand, blue and yellow are sweet, giving me the taste of vanilla when I see these colours together. Add green and it gets better, sweeter more lovely. Brown is an earth colour, it neither excites nor soothes me, but it grounds things. I taste mushrooms when I see brown, a deep, satisfying, savoury taste.

Blue, on its own, has a creamy custard taste, green is fresh like apples, red is sweet, violet is like fresh shortbread. My calculator is two shades of violet; it helps me concentrate on the maths. I did use a brown calculator, but it had orange figures on its buttons, which put me off. When I see orange I get a feeling like a migraine and a rancid taste in my mouth. However, I do like a sweet orange to eat, because I can't see the segments in my mouth. I love bananas to look at and eat. Apples need to be red only, red grapes also, cherries are good.

I have a yellow and black bicycle and I have a blue and gold bicycle with red lining, that's sweet to look at. I have an olive green bicycle, deep and satisfying to behold. I have a yellow/gold bicycle, lovely in daylight. My favourite bicycle to look at is a custom design with a crisp white frame, blue rims, green tyres, black spokes and hubs, red pedals, handlebar grips, saddle and a yellow chain. It's a sweet set of colours; I smile every time I see it.

Sweet combinations of colours exist in my photographs. Go to Flickr and look up cycle.nut66, that's my photostream. Look at thumbnails of my pictures and take in the colour combinations and the depth and saturation of colour in most photographs. Deep primary colours are all through the pictures. I seek canals and narrow boats. Narrow boats are painted in rich primary colours - I look at them, taking in the colours, and photograph them a lot. I can take the colours home with me in photographs.

People who know how orange causes me pain see my car and ask why I have an orange car. On its registration document, its colour is orange. However the actual colour of the car is caramel, a brown toffee sort of colour. Crucially, it is not orange. This is an illustration of how precisely colours are seen and how colour, or any other sensory sensitivity, are precise in autism. My car is not orange at all, and the difference is plain to me, but difficult for non-autistic people to perceive. Being autistic I see every subtlety in colour or anything else I notice in the mass of detail I can take in. Brown and orange to me are quite distinct, no matter how close they may be in colour and tone. To me they are never the same and could not be, even if other people cannot detect the difference.

I wrestled with black and white photography for years using a box camera, with some good results. I did not like the unkind comments some people made about my old cardboard camera and how I used it to make photographs; the photographs were full of feeling. The thing I struggled with was visualising subjects in black and white. I see colour and the world is in colours. This frustrated me as I tried using strongly coloured filters to turn the camera's view finder image monochrome. It helped a bit, but one needs to use different filters in black and white photography - and a strong colour is not the same as a greyscale.

The opening I needed came with a digital camera my wife bought me. I still have it and it makes good pictures. This camera has an electronic eye point viewfinder and when switched to black and white, the viewfinder shows only tones – what a wonderful device and the breakthrough I needed to do black and white photography. That viewfinder enabled me to see only tones and it was liberating as well as relaxing (colours can over stimulate and be hard on my eye when I am tired). I used the camera as peep hole to look at the world in tones and refresh my vision. Before, tones had no taste for me - instead they were inert, giving me little cognitive purchase on them. Now they have a delicate savoury taste; I can feel emotion on seeing them. My heart is happy and mind still when I see pleasing tones. I want to make them in my pictures, and park my soul a while in the pictures while viewing them.

Since being given my camera – a Panasonic Lumix FZ8 if you want to try one (it's a lovely little camera, with synergy, like all the best designs) – I look beyond the modest pixel count and see what it does. The lens, sensor and processing in this camera come together in a special way. Its pictures have a lucid clarity to them – it's simply a good design that works well and is good to use. Do we ever need more than that?

I can set the exposure to record tones exactly as I want to record them, the feel of the picture can be accurately made on a few simple controls. With time, I became used to making greyscale pictures, looking for the potential in any scene for a black and white image.

The best black and white photographs are made with silver halide chemistry on film. Try the film out and see the range and subtlety of tones it delivers, along with the brightness range it can record and the infinite variability of tone and colour it can record. Digital is all maths, electronic elements and binary code, which is good, but nowhere near as good as film. Film is art. I love the feeling as it produces an analogous representation of the scene the lens is projects - analogue photography. It does this through subtlety and the properties of the silver based chemicals in its emulsion. The photograph is made instantaneously across the whole film with no calculation or intermediate stages at all. Whatever the lens sees is recorded faithfully and simply.

My photographic goal was to record tones on film freely, with a sure knowledge of how the coloured scene I saw through the lens would translate as a greyscale. I already had the ability to see the black and white potential from a subject but could not see in black and white. Then I saw an old, Russian rangefinder camera, a Zorki 4k, in a charity shop window. It had a classic lens attached. After checking it worked, I bought it and soon afterwards loaded in an Ilford black and white film. Wow! I went straight to photographic heaven.

This old camera is slow to use and needs a degree of thought, coupled with strategic delicacy, to make a photograph. Yet when things come right, it enables the photographer and subject to relate to each other in a way that produces a soft, soulful and humane picture. Old manual rangefinder cameras are well-respected for enabling photographers to achieve these properties in their pictures.

Not long ago, I was walking the dog along the canal towpath with my son and envisaged a picture of him with our dog and the line of trees on the canalside. These elements came together in the viewfinder as I composed the picture. I thought nothing of it at the time, but I saw the scene in black and white in the viewfinder. It was more than just knowing how it would turn out, but proper black and white vision and a delight to see. The Zorki comes out with me lots now with its old lens. I can see a new thing with it. I enjoy playing with my ability to see in tones, turning the world into black and white - seeing beauty that used to be hidden under colours. It gave me confidence in myself as a person and an artist. We are all artists.

Confidence is a strange thing. Most of my life I lacked confidence. I never had much when young - life was confusing and largely inaccessible. I got told off, told not to daydream, wake up, get with it, stop being so lazy, why are you so slow? Why don't you get on with it? You useless article. You don't try hard enough. It's easy! Get along now! Stop dilly daydreaming!

At school I produced very little despite being intelligent, unable to release the potential I had. In social situations I got loads wrong - I goofed up, felt stupid, or feared the next time I would get things wrong and look silly in front of people. I tried hard, but could not tie things together, or get a handle on the situations I was in. I calculated frantically, but the gaps between my calculations and situations in real time were unbridgeable. I learned if I got things outrageously wrong people laughed and thought I was funny. That formed the basis for my sense of humour.

My sense of humour has been very helpful over the years, as I learned to act and pretend things did not bother me as much as they did. The pain would be stored up for the next meltdown. Pain and humiliation became my normal; life was spent wobbling from one humiliation to another. I tried, I really tried, and never got used to getting on with most people.

Fear was my constant companion, it still is. No matter how good I get at things fear and anxiety live in me. I am anxious and fearful right now as I write. I am at home, today has gone well, my family are downstairs and some guests are in the back room with them. I am upstairs, feeling overloaded. Someone has asked if I want to come downstairs, someone has quipped about me being antisocial. I am in fear of a difficult evening if anyone gets annoyed with me being upstairs on my own. To go down would be overload right now.

The toilet is downstairs, and to get to it I need to go through the back room and kitchen. If I do this, I will not be able to slide through and use only micro communication. People will want to make conversation. I need to rapidly make sense of the situation and deal with my overloaded senses through a fog of anxiety. If I go, I will be pressuring myself to interact. My brain will need to work in overload to make sense of what comes my way, to read people, to know who is talking to me, to work out what is being said and what is being meant. I also will need to avoid giving the impression that I am blanking anyone for fear they will get annoyed. Somehow I need to get this into a cognitive whole.

The scene as a whole takes a further load of processing. On top of processing each person, the television, the conversations, the cross talk, the body language, who is there, what they are like, recognising them (I don't remember faces and frequently get the wrong people) and having some strategies prepared for getting out of social misunderstandings and tight spots. So... I'm hanging on to my bladder, while typing, hoping I can last until they have gone and I can make it to the toilet without too much pain and overload.

In childhood this was a whole lot worse. I did not have the coping skills, knowledge and life experience I have now. However, as an adult I am still facing the same situations and processing difficulties that I did as a child. I frequently have to summon up lots of courage and use all the confidence I have gained to get on in most social situations.

The childhood pattern is repeated and reinforced in adult life. People still won't give me space for me to recollect my thoughts and reassemble processes. Then they complain that I am not up to whatever it is we are doing. Holding onto jobs has been an effort. Because I look normal and can pass for normal a lot of the time, people really won't allow me any understanding or time. In fact they are normally rude! I was talking about this with another autistic person recently, who related several bullying stories and describe the pain of appearing normal and being judged harshly when normal speech, behaviour and social norms cannot be consistently adhered to. Ouch! Life hurts. Confidence is low.

Being an adult with autism, I cannot be myself in public, as to do so would result in total social alienation and expressions of anger, even from those closest to me. Life must be a continual act.

Cycling

I've just been on Facebook, as I do several times a day. NHS Greater Manchester have put up a picture showing the benefits of cycling, including strong heart and lungs, reducing stress and buns of steel. I've had all these benefits for decades. Cycling has helped me through dark times. At my lowest, in my early 20's, cycling was one of the things that helped me stay alive. If all else failed I could ride my bike, which I did lots. I remember being at my wits' end in deep depression one day when I lived in Wales. No one was around, so I got my bike out and rode it. I kept the pace up riding along country lanes up and down hills though Hensol Forest, Welsh St Donats, Aberthin, Cowbridge, Llanlethian, Llanmihangel and Llantwit Major along the coast to Ogmore by Sea. The combination of exercise, fresh air, beautiful villages, countryside cliffs and sea cleared my pain, and I returned with enough strength to carry on for another day.

Before this, in my teens, I saw no future for myself and lost hope. Cycling kept me going for several years back then. It was the one thing I looked forward to - feeling good. Each week at school was a hideous round of not achieving, grieving for the education I was losing and feeling bad. Three events in the week kept me going: the cycle workshop on Tuesday evening and Saturday morning, and the Chiltern Hills CTC cycle ride on Sundays.

These three events gave me something I could do and be good at. I even could fix bicycles in the company of other cyclists. I was good at something. None of the club members knew how badly I was doing at school, or cared about my lack of fashion sense. I was someone who could cut it in the company of cyclists. I was good at what I did - I could build and fix bicycles very well. I could ride one hundred hilly miles in a day; I could lead rides. No one minded if I was quiet when we rode and I got the impression my company was wanted. I spent as much time on and with bicycles as I could back then.

Bicycles were my route out into happiness. I became a cycling encyclopaedia and a wiz with the tools. My bike was the best set up one in the club and I started to talk to the people that went there. They wanted to hear my opinions and some shared jokes! I had something to be proud of when I cycled. The exercise lifted my mood and gave me strength for the bad bits in between cycling activities.

I spent lots of time in school classrooms designing bicycles in my head. I used to calculate gear ratios instead of engaging with maths lessons. I could go to the bike sheds and help other students with their bicycles at break times. I rode the five miles to and from school every day, faster than anyone else could, unaware of the connection with exercise and mood. All I knew was the day would go much better if I rode fast. I got itchy legs on days I could not cycle and still do now.

Before writing today I went for a thrash on a single speed bike, taking myself to the limit three times. I buzzed from head to toe on getting home. That buzz has lasted 10 hours and is still going. I have a poor sense of my body and my balance is not great, however, on a bicycle, I can feel relaxed about my body and where it is. The bicycle provides a framework to fit my body over with five contact points. I feel connected on a bicycle; there is a lovely, warm, comfortable sense that I am an embodied being. I get messages from my body I don't feel, like I am floating somewhere nearby, watching my body from a distance.

It's good to feel like a flesh and blood human being on a bicycle. Balance gets better too, a bicycle is balanced in the same way we are balanced when walking; instead of stepping into our bodies, leaning to stay upright, a cyclist steers the front wheel into the lean to keep bike and rider balanced. Cornering stimulates my balance too. On a bicycle one leans into the bend; there is no sensation of being thrown to the side as in a car. One simply feels a little heavier, as centrifugal force combines with gravity in a fast corner. That allows my ear canals to sense my balanced without being upset by cornering forces or any such disturbance. That feels great - I can balance and walk much better after time riding a bicycle.

Cycling

Riding a bicycle outside is the most free and happy thing I can do with my body. Under the sky, my soul has freedom to go to the skies. I feel my legs are alive and my arms tremble from motion transmitted up to them from the front wheel, through the handlebars. I have hands that are controllable and work. They hold grips, pull on brake levers and click gears up and down. I feel muscles pulling in predictable rhythmic motions; I can get used to their presence and after a while I have complete control over them. My chest expands - breathing the free air fuels my body in its efforts to power the bicycle. I know where my head is and feel my neck connecting it to my shoulders that rests on my arms, which send up the familiar and comforting messages from the handlebars.

My body has a trunk that is connected to my limbs and head. It is using its muscles to brace my body and hold me over the frame. I love the feeling all this give me… because a bicycle leans into bends, my balance becomes calm and my sense of where I am in the world is a tangible reality. I fear to approach narrow gaps when walking, but would thread a bicycle through the eye of a needle without a second thought. It is a lovely feeling - to be on a bicycle and know exactly where I am and what size I am. When cycling, good ideas often come. I can pace how I cycle - slow with a gentle rhythm, or purposeful and thrash over short distances.

While writing this, my legs are tingling several hours after riding fast though town on my way to meet Joshua, my son, from his school. I rode to the point of exhaustion over no more than half a mile. I chose a single speed bike. No changing down for accelerating, just push very hard on the pedals. No changing up for speed, just spin the pedals as fast as I can. This bike allows for no adjustment of pedalling style, it's simply push on the pedals and go. I rode myself until I turned to jelly. All my adrenaline was burned off, I felt calm, my brain worked, life has been good since the ride. I will ride tomorrow and feel as good. I often ride to and at the point of pain to gives me a sense of a connected body for hours after the ride.

I ride for hours as well, slower paced, sweeter rhythm - no pain at all, just a steady flow of energy through my body with lots of time to think and to feel... to be. I sense the hedgerows whizzing by, the sky turning overhead, wheels turning, tyres rushing under the frame the road blurring under my rhythmic feet. All is in tune on these rides and I smile inside.

Sometimes I will linger on rides and feel the quiet of near silent movement. I ride slowly enough not to hear wind rushing past my ears. These are sweet tasting rides, no exertion just quiet movement. Freewheeling quietly affords moments of sweet pace. I seek these lots. When I bought the single speed bike I didn't expect to like it as much as I do. It is little more than a frame and wheels, and that is its attraction - pure, light, clean and simple. Most of all it is quiet.

Being hypersensitive to sound, I had learned to tolerate the noise of a Derailleur gear system with its out of line chain, ticking and rustling though the tiny sprockets on the gear mech. The single speed has a short chain, running a pure elliptical course round and round for as long as I pedal. It is inaudible, I even packed the free wheel with grease to silence it. I ride to meetings – sometimes across a county, there and back, taking the single speed for the relaxation, calmness and purity of the ride. I have not the words to explain the simple joy of riding this bike. It got me to my appointment and back in a sunny mood as I rode free through emerald green countryside under a clear blue sky, taking the swoops and bends in country lanes at a spirited pace.

On Sunday mornings – the day of the club cycle ride – I would be up before dawn all year round. I recall winters when the world was dark, padding around in my cycling gear going through my breakfast, sandwich and hot flask routine. I would listen to Farmers Weekly on BBC Radio 4. I liked the voices from the radio, regularly every week talking about life and growing, following the seasons, a touching place with life and reality beyond my dark little life. I got a sense there were people out there connected with life, who were growing plants and animals all year round, out there under the sky where I found my peace.

Cycling

I listened to these lives and laid my life down alongside them. Through the seasons I rode, noting every change in nature and everything that grew. These things grew alongside me; there was a common life. If I could feel this life, I could live too. It was a life beyond people's chatter and social things, the life of all things and I could pass through it on my bicycle, full of life too.

Cyclists are peaceful, eclectic people. I have always been able to find an affirmation with cyclists – possibly through their appreciation of a solitary sport – even when riding in a group. When I go places and have time to ride, I will look up local cycling groups. I went away for a couple of days in the Eden Valley in Cumbria and had a good day out enjoying the beautiful English countryside with the CTC group in Appleby-in-Westmorland.

It was like they had known me for years – cycling is a small world and there were a number of people I knew. Back in my teens it was the local cyclists that let me be me - I felt like I was someone worth knowing. Teen culture bypassed me completely, not because I let it, but because I had no means of making sense of my age peers, their ways of life, fashion and music. I did 'get' the world of cycling though, and I still do, and I like the people I meet. They are quiet methodical people.

Today, I share my weekend cycling trips with my teenage son, Josh. A gentleman at the church we attend offered us a classic bicycle, saying he had not used it for a couple of years. I like to think he wanted it to go to people who would appreciate it. Joshua and I certainly did, and painstakingly restored the bike. Josh has found out how sound a good road bike is and loves riding it. We share our faith when working on the bike and go for rides together, planning our adventure to ride the full length of Britain - from Lands' End to John O'Groats in a couple of years.

With Josh around, cycling has taken on new meaning. Sharing my thoughts, wisdom, faith and passion with a boy of my own – I am very blessed indeed. I thought I would never have a chance of living this wonderful life when I was his age. I make sure he knows exactly how much he is valued and deeply loved and has many

I Dream In Autism

possible futures available to him – that he is good enough for whatever he goes after in life. We will go together - I am not ever going to keep quiet about how proud I am of my son.

Man Watching

Desmond Morris, Manwatching, a Field Guide to Human Behaviour

My parents had a copy of this book - a large, coffee table sized edition. It contained pictures and enough text to give the information without going on too much. It was one of the first books I read. I would read it in bits, looking up the information I wanted. It had really useful chapter headings like, Yes No Signals and Expressive Gestures.

This book held a mine of information for me. My father suggested I read it, which was a good idea. It was a well set out book, full of good quality information. I'm autistic and I love accurate information. I sought answers to things that puzzled me. I hoped to learn how to interact with people. I hoped for liberation though knowledge of human behaviour. I hoped to have friends, go to parties and be able to join in with the mainstream of life. I wanted to know what to do and say, instead of being scared constantly. My fear of loneliness drove me on to find out how I could relate to people.

On reading Manwatching, I was both delighted and confused. I was delighted at the well-written, information-rich text. I read and re-read, seeking to place this information in my mental matrix for coping with life, yet this information was just that - information. Each thing sat in my consciousness like a stone. Something hard, tangible, disconnected and unusable. This puzzled me, how could having this information not help?

The trouble was that I had no way to understand, contextualise and act on the information. This is where mentoring helps - someone comes alongside another to explain and coach an individual in his or her life's development. I do not think that when I was young anyone could have helped me get this information into a form I could use. My behaviour and communication styles baffled everyone – autism was not discussed in those days.

The information widely available about autism today was certainly not available then and no one in my life would have been able to interpret it anyway. This was the late 1970s, when Lorna Wing was about to attend Hans Asperger's last lecture tour. Afterwards, she would work with her colleagues on tying findings together with further research to come up with The Spectrum of Autism and the Triad of Impairments.

I did go to see a psychologist called James Stevenson in 1978. His report, which I still have, is insightful. It describes but does not name dyslexia, a related condition. There is enough there that today could have triggered an Asperger's Syndrome Assessment for Autistic diagnosis. But the report was primitive by today's standards, and no one could unravel it further. It just added to the enigma that was my life. And the information I received became more complex and confusing, including the material I got from Manwatching.

To give you an idea of how much Manwatching did not make sense to me, I need to say something about information that is so new and alien, one has no way of comprehending it. For example, if I were to write a piece on something I understand but few readers would, how many of you would comprehend and put the information into a meaningful framework?

Let's say I were to write a piece on Sturmey Archer drivers - what would you make of it? Do you know what they are, and if I told you, could you analyse rationally via an informed mental process? I know what Sturmey Archer drivers are, and a good number of bicycle mechanics would too. A Sturmey Archer driver has nothing to do with driving cars. Did you think of driving cars a couple of sentences ago? So would you understand if I wrote an in-depth study document including findings on a Sturmey Archer driver, outlining and examining its form and function? Do you have the prerequisite mechanical understanding to make sense of an explanation? Like you and Sturmey Archer drivers, I had no means of comprehending the information in Manwatching.

All that information stood so far outside of my understanding I could not make sense of it, or even begin to make sense of it. The information sat in my mind like inert rocks. I knew it was good, but could not open the information up and use it. I would not have understood the book less if it were written in Mandarin Chinese. My teachers would have done the same with an autism evaluation report, even though it was facing them daily in their field of work, using a name like Richard Maguire.

Let's take the analogy further. If I were to show you a Sturmey Archer internal gear hub (I have a couple) and disassemble it in front of you while giving you commentary on what I was doing, do you think you would have at least a fighting chance of knowing what the driver is, understand its function, and be able to describe one without me around? And after that, would you care? Does knowing this information improve your life? It would if you were a cyclist with a non-working hub gear, or a cycle mechanic, but if you are not a cyclist, or do not have a Sturmey Archer gear hub, would you find my explanations a poor use of your time? Would such esoteric knowledge gain any traction in your life?

The knowledge about human behaviour I got seemed incomprehensible to me when I was young. However, all attempts at helping me though my difficulties back then were based on me having this knowledge, with the understanding of a typically developing child of my age. I had neither, so was not able to understand, cooperate or benefit from any help I was given. I just muddled along in depressed confusion, with cycling being my only area of demonstrable strength.

I find a lot of young autistic people are in the situation I was in. No one seems to have the understanding of their predicament and a need to help them. To do this effectively one has to have an in-depth appreciation of the inner autistic life. Not a textbook learned, shallow concept of the syndrome, or an ability to write what can be deduce from non-autistic viewpoints, but a real, 'walked a mile in their shoes' understanding.

Non-autistic people can start to learn this by spending time with real autistic people, who can train them how to see inside their inner life. I have trained many people in insights to the autistic life through explanation, exercise, practice, mentoring and reflection. My students report an amazing difference in their behaviours and effectiveness with autistic people. A lot of people say what I teach them redefines their understanding of autism and their practice changes completely.

As I said before, mentoring is valuable in helping autistic people develop a comfortable acceptance of their place in society and of themselves. Mentoring helps tie together information, consciousness and practice in the autistic life.

Oh, one last thing… if you want to know what a Sturmey Archer driver is, go to the Sheldon Brown website to find a picture of one and instructions on reassembling a Sturmey Archer hub.

Distance

As far back as I can remember I can clearly recall operating in a time and space of my own - people operated around me in their own times and spaces, where their personal experiences happened. For me, interaction was observing people and events - feeling something about them and a response from me from within my own time and space.

My reaction would be acted out, spoken, or done silently within myself. I could speak in my head; in fact I had an unusually large vocabulary from very early on. Spoken words were something I was interested in and I listened to the radio, which was on all day in our house, collecting new words to log in my cerebral database. I would say them to myself often, and repeat conversations that I could use them in. I built up strings of words and still do this ready for use in everyday life. I loved the sounds of speaking and the feel of my tongue when I pronounced them - feeling vibrations in my sinuses. I would repeat them as a matter of trial and error to see if I got the right words, sentences and intonation for the circumstance.

When I was very little this was a source of amusement to adults. Later my trial and error attempts at conversation caused criticism to come my way. I was often told that 'you should know better', 'don't be stupid', 'oh, come on', 'don't embarrass yourself' or 'be quiet if you can't say anything sensible'.

As I grew older, my speech was not seen as cute or funny. School was a horrid experience in this respect. Adults in my life and children in the street criticised me. I did not know why and tried to keep up in a world I did not understand, I tried, and I really tried. But my attempts grew further from what was required by other people. I did not know why people I had been close to as a small child became further away in culture and understanding. I knew the process was going on; I could measure it in the pain I experienced, but like trying to run through water in a dream I could not close the gap. I don't know how to describe the dawning realisation of being ostracised, except say it was deep and hollow - like being out in a vortex, seeing the people I loved outside it as I moved down to oblivion. A fear of drowning perhaps, drowning in loneliness.

Distance grew and became inevitable. I started the first year of school with a sickening acceptance of life being a sort of death - a source of nothing, a no hope. I remember my first self-harming OCD (Obsessive Compulsive Behaviour) at five years old. I began pulling hairs out. It was comforting; I could make a sensation that I could control and feel was real in all this slipping sliding, drowning and dying. The feeling was as acute as the thumps of bullies, as sharp as the pain in my heart and I had control over it. I found comfort from it, controlling the pain.

People told me I was a freak, so why not look and act like a freak? Somehow I realised that freakish behaviour was the only behaviour I could manufacture that was somehow in line with people's expectations of me. In this type of behaviour I could make a connection with past friends, albeit a hurting one. We humans need relationship to live and grow - the only sort available to me was something broken and odd. I hated it, but it was real and I needed it. It was all I had.

To be happy and part of the wider scene was what I really wanted, but knew I could not reach that goal and experienced a recurring nightmare - first in my cot and later in my bed. The nightmare was of me in my cot, later in bed, with an anvil placed across my middle. The other side of the anvil was a house, with all the people I loved in it. I could never get to the house because of the anvil. I cried out and no one heard me. I would wake in the night, in the dark, crying, frightened and alone, but felt it was no good seeking anyone out. Just as in the rest of my life I had to accept loneliness and despair at nighttime. I would lay awake, too frightened and sad to move until it was light. The coming day would be like the night, a lonely, sad and disconnected experience. Being a child I could not change or affect this – if someone had told me how to, I would have.

Top tip - give young autistic people explanations of what is happening and how they can make their lives better. We need this information as we will not guess, learn or build our own concepts of social communication. We need to be taught, this is a large part of the mentoring work I do and it's very effective.

Life with autism is something like being blind to what is happening with lots of information unsorted and not processed into a whole that can be used as a pattern for life. It's lonely in there, knowing lots yet understanding little of the life that is seen across the distance of processing and culture. I have worked with many autistic people over the years and it is like working with someone who is visually impaired. Instead the person with autism is processing impaired. Our brains swim in a sea of information, too much and unsorted.

People are perceived at a distance, calling to us over the waves of information. Of course we call back, but a lot is lost over the distance and in translation - or there is a complete lack of a basis to translate between us and them. Much of my mentoring work is giving information to all parties, so communication can happen and they can be understood. That is lovely for an autistic person. To know that there is some understanding somewhere, some, any, is good. Even the first bit of clear understanding is like a blessed and happy realisation that a relationship can happen with someone. I do not know how to tell of the joy and hope this brings to a life that up to then was lived mired in misunderstanding between us and the people we love.

Often autistic childen may seem remote and aloof. Their parents are grieving over the relationship they are missing with their children. It is lovely to help parents come to a happy realisation that the relationship they longed for is close, just a few tolerances away. I love giving these to parents and seeing hope and happiness well up in them. Even if their children are non-verbal, they will feel the warmth of love expressed by their parents coming though and conquering the distance that was there from the beginning. Inside the children there will be light, life, joy and love, welling up from all corners of their up-to-then anxious, lonely little lives. The need not have their equivalents of my anvil dreams. They can make contact with people and feel the love replacing isolation and fear. That is their basis for growing in themselves with trust and respect. It is their real seed of hope and a basis to build on.

I do not know how to express how beautiful the first contact is across the distance that was there. It's a coming into sunshine generated by a warm human life, like being touched by another life touching theirs. It's the first leap into relationship, a realisation of love and the start of hope. I have to repeat this, because of the feelings it creates in me.

Too many of us have to grow up not feeling life and its warmth. We live, we do life and we must live. Living is procedure to be done from moment to moment - what for, we do not know. Some lives have not been touched by warmth for many years. People live in the cold winter of distance for decades, existing and living out an approximation of what they see around them. The difference between that and love of life, and living it with a realisation it can be good, is so wonderful that it needs to be felt not described. I made that move in my 20's and now help people make it - by listening to them and identifying needs. By listening, I mean total, active listening, not just to the words, but listening to their souls in their quiet winter. I simply show them to the door of spring and give some simple instructions. They have their spring when they make the moves and close the distance and relate to their loved ones like they never knew they could. I do not give anyone their spring time; that would not be possible. I am simply their guide, mentor and encourager.

I can guide, as I know the way, being autistic too, and having made the journey in my life. Further to this, I teach parents and staff how to help people cross over from winter to spring. It involves giving a plausible outline for peace, focussed change of current directions and a mindful, benign presence. They will go when they are ready, but they need us to be with them.

Do You Speak Pure Human?

Micro-communication, that's what I call our autistic, finely tuned, quiet, peaceful ways of communication and body language, imperceptible to non-autistic people. Many say that autistic people don't do body language. In response, I say we do. Our body language is so subtle and minimal that people who are not autistic, and who are used to noise or more overt forms of communication and reading people, simply miss our communications.

Over three decades of working with autistic people I have grown to love our autistic ways. 'Aspie' senses (as we are sometimes referred to, which I find a positive step) are so very finely tuned - we have no need to make any form of communication, or being with other people, in any way obvious. Learning-disabled autistic people are the masters of micro-communication, relational peace and quiet ways of being with individuals.

Someone like me without a learning disability has been able to build up a set of masking skills so we appear normal in social situations. A learning-disabled person will show their autism more clearly, although they too will have done a lot of work on coping and getting on in a world where they are unusual and struggle to communicate with, and be valued by, people. We autistic people all love it when we can relax and be ourselves, and that looks very different from the things we project in public so we are accepted and can make our ways in life. I will tell you a story of how micro-communication and being purely human worked out, and how it was brought to an end by someone who did not perceive the autistic culture, communication and peace that was there.

There were three of us, autistic men. Our morning had been stressful simply from having to cope with the demands of putting on a front and behaving in ways our neurology does not equip us for - we were all putting on fronts so people would accept us. The two men with me had learning disabilities as well. Now it was lunch time and we were in a room that I had worked on to be accessible by autistic people - low stimulation, simply furnished, few colours, lots of space for ranging and using movement to calm our senses, help brains work and emotions settle. Our lunches were sandwiches.

I made the drinks as the men I was working with had been ranging (pacing) and stimming (stimulating). I use water to stim, so making drinks is a good way of accessing water for this purpose - I simply disguise my stimming, whereas the learning disabled people with me did not. They circled the room, carried stim objects and moved in ways that gave them peace. They had no fear of what I might do. We all understood each other and proceeded quietly on this understanding.

In a lot of autism services, these times would be used up with therapeutic activities and staff making a fuss, which removes the opportunity for autistic people to relax, stim and range. Being an autistic employee, I know these things usually do not work and I have not used them. They are designed by non-autistic people who are well meaning, but not autistic and do not live in our world. If I had done the more usual things with these men, they would have had meltdowns during lunchtime and would not have been ready for the rest of their day.

I train staff to be quiet and not 'busy' at all. They find this a revelation and are impressed when meltdowns cease from the people they work with. Please believe me on this, most systems for working with autistic people drive us mad and will ensure we are in pain, frightened and will melt down very soon. A mantra of mine is 'less is more' and it works every time. It gives the autistic people time to find peace and be who they are. Given time, they will come out of their protective shells and you will see the real person.

A lot of what textbooks and training courses tell you are autistic behaviours are in fact stress behaviours; natural autistic behaviour is quiet, peaceful and purposeful. Learning-disabled autistic people are in a double bind, because they do not have the articulacy or autonomy I have cultivated to help insist I be who I am in the way I live. They usually have to switch into the 'adaptive child' ego state, continually enforced by people who work with them until the next, and frequent, meltdown occurs. Then people who work with them get concerned, write up risk assessments and behaviour management plans, thus ensuring life for the learning disabled autistic person gets harder and more impossible, meltdown get more frequent and the whole horrid cycle is perpetuated by well-meaning people who send their clients to hell every day.

I see this lots and people find it a complete game-changer when I help them relax about autism, stimming and how we process our lives. I have shown staff how people they work with calm down immediately and become communicative the moment the staff begin doing nothing about autism, in the sense it is misunderstood and taught. The autistic people they work with begin finding peace and happiness in seconds of the staff calming down and taking a relaxed attitude to communication and life with their clients.

I make my living training people in autism and how to work with us. You can book me to show your organisation what the autistic life is really like and how you can succeed with us really quite simply with the right understanding, knowhow and attitude. I have no vision of being super-rich via this lifestyle choice. I simply want to help others suffering in the same situation I found myself and charge extremely reasonable rates for my services. I recall one beautiful day at a place where autistic people live and have day services.

I asked a staff team to do nothing when a frightened autistic man came into the room we were training in. Normally they would have tried to put him at ease by calling his name, asking how he is and engaging him in something. His response was always to scream and hit himself and withdraw from their company. When we all did nothing instead, he approached people, smiled and initiated contact and communication.

That worked simply because he was not being overloaded and frightened by them. He could perceive them as people in their stillness and seek a relationship with them. Some staff were moved to tears that day. That experience was so powerful that they rewrote their autism policies and ways of working for something simple relaxed and beautiful. I love it when that happens - they have learned to communicate in pure human with anxious autistic people, they have learned what I call micro-communication.

That brings me back to the lunchtime with the two men. We simply proceeded non-verbally though lunch. We communicated as three humans simply and quietly being together - in pure human, the natural autistic way to communicate. Our senses are overloaded and our processing breaks down where normal social conventions are used. We are very subtle with each other. Our senses are so acute that we communicate in almost complete silence. If you are not used to this, you might think we were ignoring each other and had no desire to communicate and relate to each other.

That is the most common misunderstanding of autistic people. In fact, we are social beings with finely tuned senses and sensing. Your 'normal' ways are too loud for us so we shut down and avoid contact in situations we fear will be painful and lead us towards another meltdown. We are so subtle that our social language is missed continually. Even researchers do not know how to look into our ways of micro-communication because they do not perceive us doing it and won't look for it. When they do come across our sensory and communication worlds they do not understand how important they are to the autistic life.

People often assume we are not doing anything and we need stimulation and motivation to get on with life. We really want to get on with life and can do this most effectively when we are at peace and in a state of emotional and sensory balance, just like anyone else. The trouble is, people think they are helping us and don't see that we are overloaded by well-meant interventions. Like Temple Grandin says, we must not be allowed to tune out, and that is a real danger requiring a careful balance between rest, down time and purpose.

The way to help us tune in fully is first to get us to a place in life where we can cope and not labour under a covering of fear of tuning in. Here again Temple has wisdom to share. She says too much attention is paid to what autistic children cannot do and not what they can do. The upshot of that is that we learn to see ourselves as faulty and lose our self-esteem and the hope and energy we need to get into and on with life.

Like anyone else, we will make huge efforts to get on in life if we feel we have the strength and self-worth to do this – and building confidence is a big focus of my work. The men I spent that lunchtime with would be happy to do all sorts of things in the afternoon if they could have their peace and stimming-time over lunch. To facilitate this I needed to do nothing other than offer myself as a benign, sensitive micro-communicative presence. And in doing so, I am also telling the men that they are good enough as they are, I respect them. I will do nothing to change them and their presence alone is good enough.

That is a powerful message to give to anyone. These men will tune in, if for a time they can be still and process in the autistic way. Remove that opportunity and they would become passive, childlike and the anxiety of dealing with that tension would drive them to meltdowns - a situation they are familiar with and wanted to avoid. So we carried on doing what may appear to be nothing. In doing this we did everything right for the time we had.

While eating, one man wanted to watch a film. He got the other man's agreement by simply picking the DVD case up and pausing a moment. The other man's stillness said he was happy with the film. In micro-communication a peaceful stillness is a good thing - it says that all is well and a suggestion is good. A tense movement or breath would indicate that something is not good. In return the other micro-communicator has read the message and will silently and wordlessly cease the activity.

As a member of staff, I communicated my support for what was suggested by being still. When something is good it simply proceeds, wordlessly. In doing that I communicated my ease at what was planned, that was picked up and understood with peace and happiness by the two men. Words would have spoiled things.

Our happiness was lovely and better than any stimulating activity that would otherwise have been foisted on them and caused them to be unready for what they wanted to do afterwards. We felt peace and enjoyed simple wordless company sharing by 'being'. That is micro-communication, communicating though sharing life. It's what I have come to know and communicating 'pure human'. A lot can be said in the silence.

What time would we get up and move from the film? The right time. When would that be? We would all know. How would we know? When we have processed and got our minds and souls ready. When we are ready we would communicate this by moving. We did not get to the stage of moving at the right time. Someone came in the room. A good person who said nothing initially - what we noticed was the sound of their clothes, shoes on the floor and the creaking door hinge. We had got to such a quiet place in our communication our senses had balanced out in the still cadence and gentle music of the film.

An autistic person is so sensitive to our sensory inputs that we pick up all we sense without filtering, prioritising or knowing if the sensory input indicates danger. That's one reason we get so anxious at sensory inputs we don't know if we are safe or not. With that in mind, take a moment to consider how frightening social situations are and how human contact can be scary. Even if you know full well that it is safe, we don't.

My coping mechanism for that is to run what is going on though my database of interactions and possible interpretations of them. That takes time and a lot of cognitive effort, one reason I shut down in social situations. I get overloaded working it all out, then I get scared, that's a common autistic experience. A learning disabled person will have a different or smaller database or maybe none at all. They will need to feel as much as possible from their senses and try to maintain composure, a difficult thing to do and impossible most of the time.

Remember what I wrote about the reaction of the learning disabled man when all the staff became still - they gave him the space and processing time to sense that they were friendly, then he could approach them. If they had been sociable in the normal way he would get overloaded, scared and run away screaming, something he did a lot.

If you work or live with a learning disabled person who runs, or freezes a lot, have a think about how scared they are most of the time and how still you could be to help them find peace and relationship. Micro-communicate with them in the quietest way possible. Deborah Lipsky in her book *From Anxiety to Meltdown* explores how to approach an anxious autistic person. She draws on her experience of being with horses, animals that are predisposed to anxiety, and how still she is with them so they can get to be comfortable with her.

Temple Grandin explores the same things in her life and work with cattle, detail focused flight animals, and draws comparisons with them and autistic humans. A calm uncluttered approach works very well. Even your breathing could be too much for an anxious autistic person. With that in mind I practice slow diaphragm breathing when with anxious autistic people, more so if they have a learning disability. This has become an essential work skill, and I teach people how to be more still than they could possibly realise so that they can find peace with autistic people.

I like it when a horse rider or trainer is in the group I am teaching because I give them time to explain how they get horses to be at ease with them. When the horse is at ease, it will trust them, and a beautiful relationship can follow. Without that trust, the horse will be too anxious for the relationship to form and it will not be inclined to cooperate at all. Many times I have heard horse riders say that they trust their horse to spot danger and get both horse and rider out of trouble. They say that can happen because they and their horse communicate by instinctive feelings, gained through mentally centring themselves to the animal, respecting the flow of movement and being guided by their horses' judgment. On the other hand, the horse trusts them implicitly after spending time watching and understanding their owner to become attuned into a partnership and will take instruction from them, including correction when necessary.

In my work I have learned to trust autistic clients. They appreciate that and become willing to venture further out into life. Should things go wrong, we simply make corrections and learn the facts and corrective routines from these incidences - there is no blame or negative judgement from me. I simply show them I appreciate their willingness to try and strength to carry on. One rule I have for myself is, don't make a fuss. The person I work with will be beating themselves up inside when things go wrong, they need me to be a strong but compassionate presence, micro-communicating non-verbally in as much peace and stillness as I can manage. Then they feel safe. And when someone feels safe they are valued.

When the calm, sensitive person entered the room we heard them like an alarm had gone off. All three of us became apprehensive in preparation for fight and flight, like a frightened stray dog in a thunderstorm. That is a normal autistic response to unexpected stimuli; we are wired up like animals, missing nothing and can jump at anything. Read more from Temple Grandin and Deborah Lipsky on this if you are interested. While I am writing this I am listening to rain sounds through headphones. The sensory reasons for this are to block out unexpected sounds that will frighten and distract me and to provide soothing predictable sounds instead so I can relax enough to concentrate.

The time we shared of quiet micro-communication had ended. We were all braced up for noise and sensory overload. That's how it goes in the autistic life a few brief times of peace in a sea of overload, which is why I have told this story. This is something everyone will overlook many of times every day causing unnecessary meltdowns. It is also important to note that the person who entered the room was sensitive and quiet by normal standards. Autistic peace is often found at levels of quiet that most 'normal' people would not notice or tune into. Autistic rest is also precise in its construction and maintenance. Our profiles are precise and fragile – like a spider's web and as finely tuned as an atomic clock.

We autistics wonder at non-autistic people and their acceptance of noise, lack of concentration and mercurial behaviour. When out in the world our experience is like being on a white knuckle ride being thrown unexpectedly from one fright to another. Out in all that noise speaking pure human gets lost, utterly lost forgotten and overlooked.

Pure human is something often crowded out by the noise and fuss of life. I see people communicate in pure human most frequently if they have profound and multiple disabilities. Their actions and communication are by necessity taken to the level of pure human. They have a talent for engaging people purely though personality and being alive in a distinct and fresh way. I find them lovely to be with and have had some good times with them. Two examples are the way they share jokes - either by responding in beautiful honesty, or by using situational humour for instance seeing the absurdity on so much of human life and interaction. They will smile from their souls up when incongruous and funny things happen in life. One needs to be tuned in to them on the purely human level to communicate and sense their communication.

I have had the privilege of training staff and mentoring many students over the years. On meeting people with extreme and multiple learning disabilities, staff and students express anxiety over their ability to communicate and are concerned that they might cause offence. My reply has always been 'just be yourself - be exactly what you are'. That is the starting point in speaking pure human. People who are different from the norm in all sorts of ways are normally very tuned in to other people. It can be a daunting experience as such people (me included) can appear to see right into someone's soul. This is unnerving as we see the potential in them to use for creating a lifeline of hope.

Learning-disabled people are good at knowing exactly how someone is operating. I often say they will strip you down to your core. It's a powerful experience and you will know if you are at ease with yourself, deep down, in their presence. My work with learning-disabled people has been useful in staying grounded and connected with people and life as it is. Get to know some learning-disabled people and let them guide you in the ways of being purely human. You will soon know who you are and how to relate to people on the purely human level in ways of peace that will astound you. Then transfer what you have learned into autism.

Being with learning-disabled people is good for us too whether we are learning-disabled or not. Non learning-disabled autistic people like me have learned a lot of fussy ways in our attempts at life and can usefully be led in the quiet ways of being purely human. We can discover our inner peace there, and if you will be still enough with us, you can help us out into the light of life. In the same way, if you are still with learning disabled people watch, learn and be impressed by their talents and energy coming to the fore, often for the first time in their lives.

In many ways I see autism and learning disabilities as cousins. Both confer a neurology and sensitive way of being human. Ways that are normally trampled on in the noise, fuss and pain of life, both need the same healing and encouragement to live life to the full.

Does Anyone Research Love?

I have been reading through more research journals on autism and saw titles bearing words like hospital, attention laboratory data, screen based multimedia use, TEEACH, symptoms, behavioural, play, serotonin, medication, bowel and on and on. I have noticed how particular research papers are, how technical they are. And then I look at autism conference agendas - they list early intervention, assessment/interaction, co morbid, secondary issues, language structure, commissioning, training, inter verbal, milestones, ABA, drugs, school, parenting and on and on. There is technical interest in autism causing lots of discussion and interest. I read nothing about love.

I was at an interview for an autism place on a committee many years ago. The first thing I was asked was 'What do you think is the most important thing autistic people need?' and I replied, 'Hope'. I think one member of the interview panel understood what I was saying but there appeared to be some incomprehension from the others. They expected me to name interventions, services and service models. I wonder what the reaction would have been had I mentioned love. I did not get that particular job.

Love is something distant and intangible for autistic people. It is hard for us to perceive if it is being shown to us. It is hard for us to project. People often accuse us of being cold. We are filled with love! Filled to bursting. Yet it all sits inside us with hardly a route out into the world. We try to show love by being reliable, doing things, being helpful and just trying to squeeze out some tender expression of love. Love can be like a grey gap between us, people, and our natural selves. We pine for loving connections within and without ourselves.

Living on the inside of this gap in a cold little world, we hear people around us saying critical things in relation to our ability to love and relate to each other. They even ask each other if we know what love is! They say we have a reduced capacity to love. Some say we cannot receive love. Yet inside we reach for love, we yearn for love and our hearts are breaking. The suffocating grey in our life closes in on us. The love is pushed deep down and away from what we are conscious of. We become increasingly conscious of pain, sadness, pain, pain and more pain. We walk in despair taking small painful steps in the darkness and we still hear people criticising us from the outside. We retreat further and the criticism becomes louder.

We grow, we long to love. We live in an uncertain world where we are not sure that our parents love us. Our 'normal' siblings add to the confusion, noise and meltdowns. We hear from schoolteachers that we are not developing properly. Things are done to help us develop. How do we develop when we don't really know who and what we are? How does learning and development happen in a stunted, grey life where love is not touched? We get more messages about how we are not coping. We know this already. Our emotions are anxiety and sadness. We become familiar with being self-critical as it's all we learn. Self-criticism may be our only link to people and our souls. A life of common and confirming criticism is at least real and tangible. A stunted relationship is better than none.

Just like non-autistic people we crave relationships and fear loneliness. Yet we live a terrified state, afraid that the tenuous critical hurting relationships we have may end, possibly in the next meltdown when we learn we have annoyed our parents again and make people distant from us. Our world suddenly becomes a darker grey. Love is now a distant dream, no, not even a dream – it must not be dreamed of, desired or hoped for. To want love or to continue to believe it can be felt becomes a cruel tease from within our souls. Hope of love must be extinguished to relieve even that pain that a hope for love will bring. We only have strength for the pain of a grey, isolated, meltdown sort of life. We cannot carry the hope of love.

We grow, we don't speak, we don't look we survive. We keep on through grey tedium and negative messages. To think positive is another cruel tease from within. It daren't happen. To have a positive thought or to have aspirations is a hurt too great to bear.

People still look at us and say we are not developing. We dare not develop. We have extinguished hope after extinguishing love. We are gawky, unlovable teenagers by this time. Depressed to within an inch of our lives, yet still alive.

There is a dark hopeless way of living, beyond tears inside hopelessness. Life will still be lived, just. Life, a thin life, a life where people express more concern, educators say things are not working. A life where the word 'lazy' is used more and more in regards to us. Where anxiety boils over into meltdown with sickening regularity. More interventions are named; all fall short of being any help. The basis for success is not present. Where is the self-esteem, hope and feeling of being loved? These things did not work in the past for the same reasons.

There will be memories in my mind of small successes - the learning of YuGiOh strategies and trading of cards, but friends eventually grew out of them. The front door lock was fixed one morning, the autistic perseverance and problem solving was used to dismantle, repair and rebuild it - that got some thanks. Mum's computer got a virus and I fixed it - a bit more thanks. Sister's boyfriend's car broke and distributor is fixed - thanks given.

A little hope of being accepted by peers surfaced, but social skills were not up to the task. We cannot make the most of these openings, so hope fades again. We've un-jammed the toaster so many times but dad became angry when the toaster was disassembled. He would not listen to my plea that if the right adjustments were made it would not jam again and I get told off. No one seemed interested that the 29-degree pitch on the roof was too shallow and that a 38-degree pitch would work better.

Other people seem not to notice these important things. Thus possibilities for relationships and talking about interesting things cease. Anything we are good at, or interested in, gets lost in incomprehension and criticism for other things that do not make sense to us. People seem to ascribe more meaning to how we behave socially than we do. But what we do is often our only means of being noticed and therefore... liked.

Time rolls on, adulthood looms. Fear of being utterly rejected by family. A conviction that love is absent. A sickening fear of the end of teens and where twenties start, still no hope. Other people are observed getting on in life. Loves are found, relationships are formed. Aspirations turn into careers. Life for people moves. The autistic life is still in childhood with the hope removed. The years number twenty or more. What is life now? The head droops, shoulders curve, and my pain goes from grey to black. The sun shines too bright and shows too much. A tired, dusty bedroom must suffice. Suicide seems an attractive painkiller. A cessation of this knotty horrid little life is a relief.

But life will continue in most cases. There is still one little morsel of interest to be had at a time. The development of televisions might prove interesting, along with technological and social developments in television. Programming and internet TV provide a little relief. Channel fragmentation and viewing figures give interest as do channel dwelling and hopping. Wood grain reproduction holds an interest for a time. The 43 average numbers of dendritic rings on a wood floor tile seems interesting. A study of trees and their ecology holds interest and staves off suicide.

Next comes an interest in spoiler profiles on cars along with the effect they have - side wind stability becomes interesting. All cars in the town are observed and assessed for side wind stability and rear window cleaning systems are scrutinised. Cars on the road become like friends showing themselves and their forms for scrutiny and a relationship of sorts.

People would be better, but they are too unpredictable and eventually incomprehensible. A police officer notices the autistic person checking out cars, becoming suspicious that cars are being checked prior to stealing them. Questions from the authoritarian figure mean that an unbelievable, but truthful, answer follows: the side wind factor is interesting, really. He is not convinced by this.

The lack of eye contact and slowness in answering questions is taken as being evasive. An arrest follows, then a meltdown on being taken to the police car. Then restraint is used and a van is called for. No one believes us anymore. Then we retreat back into our grey world of disconnection. Following this we don't go out again. Interests are lost a grey life turns to black. A deeper uncertainty and loss of hope follow.

The road to hell is paved with good intentions. I have seen this in my life and the lives of nearly every other autistic person I have met. This is I why asked if love has been researched. So often we are seen as people, to be fixed, to be therapy-driven into a normal line of developmental milestones. We hear all about the things we do not do and the milestones we miss. I know parents, therapists and educators spend lots of time discussing us, measuring us and seeing this within negative frameworks. Guess what message we get from this? We believe that we are substantially wrong and not good enough. Remember we are literal thinkers and will literally believe these things when people talk about us in this way.

This is the story I have told and it unfolds in too many of our lives. I so often see, and am asked to help, young autistic people in the situations I have described. They hate themselves, dare not feel love and live grey sad, hurting lives. Specialist interventions and services are tried and people are often left wondering why no progress is made. Then negative reports are made about failures and partial successes. Pause a while and take in what this is doing to people's self-esteem and the confidence parents have in their parenting abilities. What does this do for the flow of love and self-esteem? The road to hell is paved with good intentions.

I have met more depressed autistic people in their late teens and early twenties than I can remember. The story is usually like the one I have told with individual variations. The other significant part of the story is a mother who has guessed more of what is going on than anyone else has realised. A mother in pain over her autistic child who so wants to love her child in a way she feels is adequate. That mother can no more bridge the love gap than her autistic child can - no one has shown her how to bridge this gap.

Instead she has been shown or sold therapies and interventions of varying quality and relevance to her child and these may only have worked to a small degree.

I meet and read of mothers who grieve at the regression they see in their autistic child. As the years go by, their child stops smiling, talking, trying. Then lots develop depression and attempt suicide.

I have helped pick up too many young autistic adults whose self-esteem and feeling for love have been quite extinguished by 19 or 20. They stumble their way through life from one interest to another stimming (stimulating) and self-harming on the way. Parents wring their souls with grief and guilt in the background. I use my own survival and success experience in my work. I too am a parent of an autistic child. I have been so careful not to let him be damaged on his way through life. He needs every piece of self-esteem, hope and love he can grasp, having only a distant awareness of the testing and techniques so often used on autistic children.

He knows about love though. And he knows what he is good at and why people like him – because Julie and I tell him. We make it clear for him to see and feel good about himself. We encourage positivity, however small, however often. And we show love through different channels – be that quiet time or micro-communication or spoken and written words full of pride delivered with love.

I my work I show autistic people and their parents that they are good, they really are. I do not patronise. That would be spotted miles off by a nervous, hurting autistic individual and would make the situation ten times worse. I genuinely see the good in all people and know that to develop in life we need to feel good. Getting through to this in a depressed autistic world is not easy, or a task that can be wholly completed. There are so many autistic adults in life whose default understanding of themselves is self-critical and complements are hard to register. Self-doubt and pain is ingrained in all of us to the deepest places in our souls. Love helps us out into the light of life.

Does Anyone Research Love?

Please research the usefulness of love.

Geworfenheit

Geworfenheit is a word used by Martin Heidegger to refer to being in a situation not of one's choosing or control. I heard Geworfenheit first on the radio on a book review programme on BBC Radio 4, collecting words from voices without faces, voices of the world, travelling with them in their speech. Geworfenheit, it stuck, it goes straight to the heart of being autistic; to be in a world not of one's choosing, a world one does not understand, a world viewed from a distance with distortion of senses, perception and understanding. A world one does not belong to, a world beyone reach which has to be sensed and touched remotely with little comprehension and with a good deal of fear.

A world that does not understand the autistic person's attempt at getting to know it. Where people's sounds and actions are repeated with a tentative, autistic understanding, voice and touch. In return there comes criticism, distance, an absence of understanding and reproach.

Like a hermit crab I pop into my shell. I still view the world around me and the 'shadow people' who tell me off say I'm silly, funny stupid and worse. Like a hermit crab I carry a shell, one you cannot see, one that weighs heavy on me, one I must build stronger and repair every day. It is the place my soul goes to during the day. It is a place removed from the physical sensory world, apart even from my body.

I live in my shell, it's not physical, and it is real. In there is protection for my soul. I remember our second house - I was three or four. I remember the window at the front, the stairs to the right and the shelves with things on them. The shelves were where I would look when people were there, they were the things that didn't move. I watched them, settled and travelled with my soul away from people. That little sheltered place outside of me where I lived, watched and if I felt confident I would venture to contact people.

Outside of my shell my body moved, it got shouted at, bullied and hurt. In my shell I felt this remotely, it hurt less in there. My shell has served me well from then, to starting school to today. I still use my shell as I did then. I choose when I come out, not often. I can act and drive my body through life, I have more routines now, my shell has more facets and it's still the one I made in that house long ago, by the stairs in front of the shelves aged three or four.

I try to model understanding and accept my shelled place in the world, I touch it now and then. My shell is mine - I travel through life in it, a comfy slipper for my soul. I won't tell you when I step out, because that could hurt too much. A hermit crab won't come out when it senses movement above and nor will I. So I send my body instead.

I join my body to touch the world now and then. When I ride free on my bicycle, when I lead worship, when I am with my son, when I am in prayer, when I am in the cloak of night - but just quickly so not to risk hurt.

I live by a Geworfenheit state in the world - not because I set out to do this but because I learned to decades ago, when I began to reach out to people before I knew that hurt.

Help Your Children To Know Their Possible Futures

As autistic children grow up, we develop much later than children of our age and it gets more apparent when we get to our teens, becoming critical in early twenties. One huge thing in all this is anxiety about our future. We grow up being told we are faulty - our autism is described as a problem, so we think we are problems. The resulting effect destroys our self-esteem and confidence, consequently increasing our rates of depression, suicide and underachievement.

Most of this can be prevented by first seeing autism as a positive. We have special brains and ways of living. We see more deeply than other people and specialise in what we are passionate about. Life would not be what it is without us; we are the people who see outside of the box. We are the inventors, innovators and people of deep sight. Our ways of knowing life and how it works drive many of us into caring roles: nurses, doctors, carers, social workers, teachers, therapists of all kinds, caring, policy and campaigning.

We make good campaigners - we see things that need attention and our drive will get us through a lifetime of making things better for people. We like social justice and ecological issues very much.

Just about anything that works, from cutlery to computers, aeroplanes and ships, will have a significant autistic input. We can see sense and analyse complex systems and engineer them well.

We do not mess around and play politics although we do get into Politics with a capital P, because of the things we will campaign about.

We like and are good at pursuing our specialist interests. These are ways we can get into employment. Through that employment we have a good chance of making friends and meeting our life partners.

Yes, we are socially awkward and don't always say the right thing. We can be withdrawn and give cause people to believe we have little talent and ability. But get us tuned into our passionate interests and you will see abilities way above expectations – as we are able to link other things into our passionate interests. We are hardworking and persistent. We don't get bored easily when we are on a mission. If you want a project doing - hire an autistic person whose passionate interest is connected to that task then watch in delight as it gets done – diligently and swiftly. A lot of us are high achievers because we can do something well - often it's only one thing such as computers. (Bill Gates is a famous example.)

A top tip when employing an autistic person is not to make us try to multi-task and multi-role since we are specialists (although we will do well at other tasks if they can be linked and interspersed with our specialities). If we are expected to be generalists and be equally competent to a shallow level in several areas, we will cease to be effective. We cannot maintain interest at anything less than complete involvement – that's why we will not function well, or for long, if we cannot do the things we are very good at for extended periods of time.

I was given the task of setting up an autism and learning disability specialist service within a wider service. My dedication and enthusiasm for the work was limitless. I ensured that all the staff were trained properly and ready for all manner of work. I kept the team together, told them they were good, mentored them on how to behave with individuals suffering from autism and backed them up. That was a rewarding time in my working life because of the positive results we produced in the lives around us.

Then things were reorganised and new management introduced, who did not value what I did and pressured me to work differently through multi-roling. They would not be persuaded of the service I provided and a lot of it was taken away from me. Things went badly after that. I simply could not meet the demands being made of me, or deal with the negative sensory overload and uncommunicative environment I was expected to work in.

Today, I am employed as a freelance mentor and public speaker in the field of autism. People hire me in for specific autism-related issues. What I do works well with responsive impact and I get more assignments that involve mentoring. I help young autistic adults see their talents and to accept their autism as a neat way of getting on with an interesting life. I have followed the careers of happy successful autistic people and there is one common theme - they have all followed their passionate interest to become successful because they are very good at it.

In a video on YouTube, Temple Grandin advises young people to be 'super good' at what they are good at. She is also right in what she says about us not being able to play workplace politics and I too advise autistic people to stay out of workplace politics. However, employers will want us for being good at something the employer needs and we will feel good about being able to fulfil that need.

Young autistic people pay a lot of attention when I tell them of the possibilities for them to succeed in adult life. Always give possibilities (plural), because if only one is given and it does not work out they will be stuck, stressed and unable to see another way forward. Lots of young people have not heard this before - they listen to words about their deficits, problems and social shortcomings. So when I tell them ways they can make futures for themselves they go into deep thought and exhibit peace and a latent purpose.

Parents too feel better knowing that there are ways their autistic child can succeed in life as they are rarely told the possibilities. They like hearing this news from an autistic person who is happy in adult life – one that has had to solve many of the problems and challenges to overcome deep despair.

I never claim life will be easy; I don't think it's that simple for anyone. Being autistic means we have more difficulties to overcome with fewer social skills to influence people. I repeat the effort needed - like Temple Grandin said we need to be 'super good' at what we are good at and that means a lot of hard work in all areas of our lives.

We stand a much better chance in life and work harder if we feel good about ourselves – that applies to us all. I was delighted recently, when talking to a group of sixteen plus students about life beyond education, to find a lot of them felt good about themselves. What they wanted to know is how to succeed and get an idea of their possible futures. They wanted to have routes shown to them so the darkness beyond education could be illuminated and followed with focus and determination.

They liked hearing this from someone who had tested these routes and could report on their effectiveness. They wanted things explained in autistic details and advised on what actions to consider when things went wrong. They wanted guidance on resilience, handling meltdowns, dealing with setbacks and not giving up on hope. The same works for adults too. Often we are unable to make much progress in life socially, personally and with work. We are stuck in a holding pattern, feeling bad and seeing no way to a bright future. Adults can initiate and take their lives forward if they have the confidence and a plan. This can take time, especially building the confidence needed to achieve even a small success. In all this there is one huge autistic advantage to be used in a strategy - we are focused, persistent and unlikely to give up once we are on a mission. These qualities are often what help us to succeed.

An autistic child is made for an atypical life. It's good to know just how special we are and it can be fun if embraced properly. Although it will be hard work and require constant persistence, be prepared to pay little attention to what is expected of development in normal terms. We develop in the autistic way, which will mean social and emotional development will be at least half their chronological age when viewed from the non-autistic viewpoint. Development is spiky and inconsistent, but that's normal in autism and part of our specialist way of life. We do not normally show any rounding out of our development before thirty, usually later. We need to feel good about being autistic.

Autism will not go away, it is part of who we are and we need to feel good about it so we can be at peace with ourselves and have happy lives.

Parents, please help your children to believe these things and feel good about your parenting. By the way, statistically, there is a fifty per cent chance you are autistic too and you have applied yourself to life very well to get where you are. You will have succeeded without a diagnosis or any help and that is good on your part.

Here's One I Made Earlier

The 'make and do' demonstrations on the long running BBC children's TV programme Blue Peter were a fascination for me. When I was growing up it was essential twice-weekly viewing. Back in the 1970s the presenters - John Noakes, Val Singleton and Peter Purvis - introduced millions of children to interesting things in the studio and screened films they made out and about. Once a year they would go to another country, somewhere really different to report about life there.

A huge part of Blue Peter was the 'make and do', where the presenters showed us how to make things, all sorts of things, accessories for toys, useful things like desk tidies, art and cooking. Blue Peter was broadcast live and un-prompted back in the 1970s. What we saw on our screens was happening in the studio in London in real time as we watched it. So the 'make and do' could be shown from beginning to end on the show - there was no time for glue to set or things to cook - the presenter used the immortal set of words 'and here's one I made earlier'. After sticking things together, they reached under the counter for one they had made earlier. When demonstrating cooking there was a cooker on the set to supply 'one they made earlier'. I loved this system of keeping going through a live presentation by being pre-prepared with things made earlier.

I struggled through my childhood with disconnection and loneliness as my constant companions and started thinking about the 'one I made earlier' approach. Most of my life, then and now, happens in a stream of events that I am not prepared for and have little or no understanding of until I can consider them and work things out. When I have things worked out, of course, the moment has passed and my response is out of date by seconds or days. The reason I was quiet as a young boy was because I had no bank of responses.

I don't know when I started doing it, but I was aware that I could 'make one earlier' in regard to speech for use at some time in the future when the need arose. These TV demonstrations depicting pre-made items were useful for any situation I could imagine and applied to conversational situations or mannerisms for me. I laid down sound tracks of words to use, thousands of them - I have them now and have added lots more to the sound library in my head along the way. I have also pre-prepared a series of actions to go with the words, or actions on their own for just about anything I do. This technique is so useful that I run most of my life on things I prepared earlier, it's a wonderfully free and efficient way of coping - being able to act in the world and get on with people.

Hope Transfusions

Sometimes someone's self-esteem is so low, I do what I call a 'hope transfusion'. This involves coming alongside them and transfusing hope from me to them simply by being close to offer lots of encouragement (even if it means using micro-communication tactics) and ways to deal with their situation. Afterwards, I am utterly exhausted but the exercise is worthwhile and proved positive in rescue cases of extreme anxiety and hopelessness.

I Am Alive When I Am Speaking And Teaching

Yes this is a chapter.

The white space below indicates how I feel when I am alongside someone mentoring them. It's an incredibly fulfilling quest. Their future is bright...

I Dream In Autism

Please read this chapter while listening to 'Love Song' by the Utah Saints.

I was lying in bed on a morning several years ago, staring at the swirls of plaster on the ceiling. As usual, I remembered a dream. My dreams are full of people and the interactions I have with them. They are mostly set in a scene of holidays, not real ones, but ones based on reality with a significant twist. People I know well are in the dreams, being who they are in real life, but acting strangely different. The difference being that I am communicating freely with them, and their behaviour is very odd. They are subject focused just like me, but I can work them out and get on freely without the normal struggle to keep up and understand.

The holidays in my dreams are different too. As a family we go to Holy Island in Northumbria - an island with access by road at low tide. In real life the causeway is about three miles long, but in my dream it's thirty-two feet long and has been like this for years. In the dream it floods to eighteen inches and stops traffic. In real life it gets a lot deeper, with strong currents stretching over a half-mile, needing a bridge and refuge box for anyone stranded. The south of Holy Island in my dreams has a long road up and over soft downlands with beautiful cliffs and a small bay with a cafe in it. The road and downs are usually misty and I do not always get to the bay. The real Holy island has the causeway road, but this runs next to sand dunes; there are no downs or cliff. I am telling you this because I am autistic. I want to tell you this information. In my dream I am 'normal'.

The village in my dream is like Baile Mor, the village on the island of Iona. Iona Abbey is also in my 'dreamlike Holy Island', but much smaller, and the cloister buildings are some way off. We stay in rather strange holiday cottages, and sometimes can't quite get to them. I try to go down to the village to see the tide cover the causeway and get lost or waylaid. The jetty for the ferry on Iona is in the village, but on my Holy Island the village is a long way from the causeway, which means I do not get to meet my family - we are separate in the dream, which is troubling and I wake up feeling sad. We have also been on holiday in a caravan in my dreams (we never have in real life). The caravans in the dreams are always unusual in their layout and we don't get to stay in them but instead tow them around. I check pitches and that's it. I travel such a lot in my dreams and the details of travel are central. I don't quite get anywhere though, except for places unexpected but they do not have a real feeling about them and I am always one removed from people - like being in a goldfish bowl. I can travel in real life yet people are removed in my dreams.

Somehow, I have meaningful relationships in my dreams with opening gambits in conversations and can 'hold my own'. People talk to me and like me, using subject-based discussions without small talk. They take long periods of times to be quiet between speaking and have animated action when talking. Yet I am still removed in my goldfish bowl world, just like I am in real life.

Right now, I am listening to 'Sun' by the Utah Saints. There are repeated sampled vocals that are more rhythmic than comprehensible. They are distorted at first then one can discern 'Grey sky in one direction. Clear blue sky in another direction'. Repeated again. Then there is another lyric I cannot hear very clearly. The music rises like a sunrise and the last words are 'everything looks kind of ok', allowing a feeling of reassurance to escalate from the word to everything in the melody. The whole effect is inexplicable, yet rooted in something physical and discernible - a change in the weather. That is so like my life and dreams. I want to have a clear result but as in life the result is unfathomable. My dreams do not come to conclusions, the journey continues.

Dreams are clear yet unreal, literal yet impossible.

I have to spew this feeling out into words for you to feel my confusion and constant analytical spherical existence. Like life... so like life, that I did not stop to think about them but when I did, I saw no disjunction between dreams and waking life. Waking and sleeping just followed on in a procession of goldfish bowl reality.

Disjuncture and absence of cohesion - no place in the world for me, I am separate and in my bowl.

Waking life is spent continually observing, computing, running videos in my head - seeking places of connection in a synthesised, repetitive visual and sensory world. Real places being perceived in fragmented ways, in-head videos and imagination filing in the blanks. People entering and disappearing - becoming fleetingly discernible through the distortions of the thick curved glass of the bowl, yet I am not able to touch them through the glass. They look at me and I can see their quizzical faces – it's the sort of face I can recognise, as I have had a lot of practice. That face happens before they leave after dealing with me, or worse...

In my dreams the worst does not happen except for a sense of alienation, which is often worse than a definite bad outcome. Life is to be lived on the outside disconnected from the inside. I sense and do not compute. People fade and I am alone again. People become wisps - real but distant and unintelligible. I get better at discerning people with experience. I can put down more templates for speech, affect, mood and behaviours. I can compute more and make more connections but further connections are elusive.

There really is no huge difference for me in dream or waking life. I do dream in autism.

In All This Confusion There Are Tangible Benefits

In a life containing mostly confusion and enigma, tangible and understandable things are a definite necessity. They are enjoyable - they give grounding, add fun and allow for mental exercise - something I can connect myself to people with.

My absolutes have normally been technical, making mind maps for understanding people, systems, emotions, politics or things. These things are bliss when I can catch on to them and suddenly I am in a reverie. I do not connect on an overt level well unless there is some tangible and definite thing to connect to. I know most people greet in all sorts of verbal and non-verbal ways on meeting. Being autistic, I want to connect using micro contacts and communications on a silent spiritual level. Neuro typical people do not perceive these micro greetings and communications. They say I am quiet and want to compensate by talking.

I appreciate the kind motives behind this, but it sends my mind into a tailspin of overload. I try to do a passable impression of a normal response to the greeting. It often comes out quiet and stilted. Then the person greeting me becomes concerned, confused, or put off by my inadequate response. From there on in, the interaction is usually beyond saving on my part and I go deeper into overload. I know that certain facial expressions and eye contact is necessary, and can just about do these, but I am in no way able to say anything appropriate. All my cognitive systems are screaming for respite from this situation. Inside, I am feeling sad that things have gone wrong again. The other person usually feels rebuffed and does not usually initiate communication again.

In all this angst I need absolutes, something I can focus my mind and speech on. I also need time to process and recover using considered responses. I love company and friendship but I cannot do these things in the normal way. I think appearing normal and being obviously intelligent works against me in social contacts. I

135

see people being surprised, I see the confusion and discomfort at my inability to maintain dialogue beyond a few sentences. My processing has been working so hard that I run out of brain energy and quickly drop out of conversation. People find this hard as I appeared so normal a few seconds ago.

I need things to hold on to in interactions - things I can process. They give little rests from the fuzz of life and processing it all and when I have them - they are sweet and good.

Keep On Keeping On

I am by inclination logical. I feel lots and over the years, worked hard on getting in touch with acting on feelings, mainly in response to my wife - her needs and what she has taught me about the world of feelings.

By nature, I am a doggedly persistent person and have always had an unrelenting characteristic of just keeping going no matter what. I keep going when I can only see a little ahead, or there is no view of the way forward. During my darkest years I have refused to accept defeat and instead kept on and on... and on. This attitude has kept me alive.

It does not seem logical or possible for me to give up on life and now I feel it flowing very strongly within me. My life has been battered and tested lots. It does not stop. The thought of stopping does not compute, I can't stop. I could not stop even at my lowest. I would go for just one more day, or a night or hour or from event to event. Even when I have felt paralysed by depression, incomprehension and seen no course of action I have just clung to existing. The thought of not existing can't happen in my mind. I will live. Even when being bullied as a child I just kept on going. When at my most depressed I let the pain accompany me - hoping I would find one thing, no matter how small, to hold on to. It would be a thought, a fantasy or an action.

These thoughts would be analysing aspects of life, observation I made, working through technical understandings or trying to make sense of people. My mind would turn over like a tumble dryer, turning thoughts round and around. I considered them again and again from the same angle, and then I tried other angles. I call this process going on a thought safari. I want to know how far I can go and what synthesis there is with other thoughts, subjects and areas of enquiry. I would consider things technical as well as culture and behaviour.

I saw behaviour as something other people did, as I had no system of referencing this to my own actions and understanding of the culture around me. I would also spend hours analysing technical systems. I can visualise these. I would spend time looking at cars and I did the same for aeroplanes, ships, steam engines, windmills, tractors, farm machinery, bicycles, kitchen utensils, lawn mowers, power stations, jet engines, model aero engines. Citroen cars with their mechanical quirks, computers, clocks and watches, cameras (I love cameras, I've got a huge collection of them, I know how they work and just how to use them to best effect), motorbikes, drills, models and lots more. These mechanical and systematic worlds were lovely places to go to in dark times.

I even thought of ways to improve things. I used to write to Raymond Baxter, when he presented the BBC's popular science programme 'Tomorrow's World', with sketches of my ideas. He always wrote back with an informed analysis and genuine technical criticism. He introduced me to friction and thermal losses in mechanical systems, something I have held on to ever since. This is one reason why my car is in such good condition since I know all the ways it can lose energy, over and above the massive thermal losses inherent in piston engines.

Most power goes out through the exhaust pipe in hot gases that have done nothing to propel the car. My current car is a Nissan Micra; its engine was designed to minimise thermal losses through flat top pistons and combustion chamber roofs that are as near hemispherical as the designers can get. All its bearings are designed for low friction and use lighter weight oils than previous engines used. I keep the tyres at optimum pressures and drive to brake as little as possible, consistent with safety. I get 53mpg out of it on a run. It's all to do with energy conservation and minimising losses. Even keeping the car clean makes a difference – yes, really, I have read the science.

By the way, I know I have been on a diversion in the last paragraph - I went with it as it illustrates something of my autistic mind in action. I find concentrating one subject, when in deep thought, difficult. But my thought safaris go to all kinds of places. Just let me read a textbook, a research paper, a copy of *New*

Scientist or have a conversation with someone who knows something about something that adds to my thought landscape and I'm off on deliberation safari pretty quick. I model and play with the new information, morphing and synthesising all this into a massive consciousness I have of system, culture and the way things go. I love reflecting on how human culture shapes the things we make, our priorities and our attitudes. All this is so exiting I cannot let it go. It is a huge fuel for my life and motivation to keep going. And usually this thought process is happening as someone is waiting for an answer – staring at me.

I also do things, lots of things. When I was younger I used to make models. Collect and run model steam engines. I ran these lots. I would oil and clean them and make them run as efficiently as possible. I love watching mechanical systems at work. I also learned how to build and maintain bicycles. I understand the synergy and efficiency needed in a good bicycle. I haven't built a bicycle for a few years but I maintain the ones I have meticulously. I ride nearly every day. The bikes I have are unusual and great to ride. If you have already read about my passion for bikes in another chapter then please forgive me as I repeat myself but that is also a characteristic of the autistic mind. I have to tell you things repetitively to ensure you understand. I love tinkering, making cars and bikes go even better than they already do. I have an old car and it is in better condition than it was when I bought it. I know all its bits. I surf the web looking for advice on preservation and maintenance.

I collect cameras and use most of them whenever I can. I clean and keep them ready for use, carrying a camera everywhere with me - to meetings, to schools, to supermarkets. I take pictures daily. I observe and record. I research the cameras. I study photographers' work and techniques. I also have a visual way of seeing and comprehending the world. Photography is perfect for how I see and perceive the world around me.

Since leaving school, I have spent more time studying than when I was at school. I am a qualified preacher, I retook my school maths exams and went on to achieve health and safety qualifications along with a degree in theology and religion. I wonder if the people that bullied me achieved their life purpose. I sincerely hope so and forgive their ignorance.

A colleague said to me that I could not possibly do nothing without it resulting in something. She was right. Whether in thought, action, or more usually both at the same time, I keep on learning and synthesising ideas. All of this comes from a drive to be positive. In my own quiet way I used to spend most of my childhood time working things out, fixing things and carrying on because to do nothing felt bad.

Within all this thought, whizzing around my head, I have spent considerable time weighing up evil actions and all the things that degenerate our human condition. This comes from my experiences of being bullied and discriminated against. Cruelty simply does not make sense to my logical mind - evil dehumanises both the people who believe and carry it out and the people it is directed at. I worked this out at a very young age as a frightened boy, ridiculed for being different. Evil cannot have a positive outcome, it is seated somewhere very dark in the human psyche. It cannot develop anything new, nor can it make new life. Instead, it succeeds in only degradation and death. The only logical way to carry on in the face of evil is to be positive, to love, to build up, to grow and nurture. I found this applicable to any system, people and place in time.

I tried to work out what goes on in the minds of people who do evil - something that is alien to my autistic mind. As far as I can see, evil comes from some sort of anger – a need to pervert good processes and the reward is self-affirmation of something or someone, putting them down and feeling powerful on top of this ugly situation. When the bullies attacked me I could see them getting some sort of satisfaction from their actions. And because so much life grows around them, evil people seem to have an inexhaustible source of things and people to hurt. Evil invents nothing but itself, it can have no life or fertility outside of its own inward looking and warped view. It only has sustainability because of all that is good. If there were no goodness in the world an abundant life of evil could not operate as it is a self-deluded and self-serving system feeding on all that is good.

I love life, kindness, humility and all that is good; I really, really do. This is also a major reason for my Christian faith. In Jesus I see someone thoroughly good, the author of life and all that makes life worth living, coming up against evil in all its forms. Refusing to compromise and being murdered on a cross for being true to God and all that is good. As someone who has been misunderstood, bullied, disadvantaged and hurt lots in life, I see a friend in Jesus, someone who will affirm and encourage all that is good. I also see his resurrection as the most positive affirmation of the indestructibility of God's life and the life he put into everything. In the company of Jesus, I keep on keeping on going, even surer of the value of life.

My faith is based on logic and a logical love of life. Through many hard knocks I have learned that to cling to life is the way forward in even the darkest of times. To lose hope is to lose my hold on life. I will not compromise with or practice evil, it offends my very being. I just don't see the point of evil. It has tried to degrade my life, it succeeded to some extent but life is stronger.

Today, being logically positive is the main reason for carrying on in life. Yes I do get hurt. I do get annoyed. I do feel anger. I do use strong language at times. There are times where I wonder if the way forward is totally obscured. I just hold on and keep going.

I do not give up on things once I have set my course. I may take breaks, they may take a long time, but I am determined. I have had to be determined. Success in life has come hard. Years ago I cried when my dreams of university and a degree faded in front of me. I saw a life of sweeping floors for a living, loneliness, and the frustration of not achieving anything like my academic potential for the rest of my life. The dream of a degree never entirely went away and by a circuitous route I did get to go to university. I was not in a degree course originally. Then the opportunity came for me to use my existing credit towards degree status - I went for it, and eight years later I graduated from Oxford Brookes University at the ripe old age of forty-three!

Today I have completely reversed the situation I was in at nineteen and a no hoper. It took decades, which were not at all easy, but I just kept on going.

All this does come from a deeply autistic part of me. Well, all of me is deeply autistic. Autism is an intrinsic part of me, it's everything I feel, think and do. There is not another way for me and I'm fine with that these days. It's hard work but this is the hand I have been dealt in life. No use complaining, although I do, sometimes it is somewhat cathartic. I will use what I have and go on with life.

Being logically positive is the way I approach my work with autistic people. I naturally have a positive view of people. Problems are to be worked through; logically there is no other way. Life carries on. What else can it do? I work alongside people and their families in an analytical problem-solving sort of way, remaining optimistic throughout. Someone with low self-esteem (like lots of the people I work with) needs someone who is positive about them and has a 'can do' attitude to sorting out the problems they face. They need to be believed in, just as I did. Often my team and I are the first paid people they come across who do believe in them. An unconditional positive regard is essential in our work, and is one of the first things I help people to value on starting their journey to happiness.

Don't get me wrong - I have been to the pits of despair, lived through this and climbed out of that. I will never forget the pain. But life these days is better, knowing I have been teased to the edge of destruction. I know my limits and what my strengths are.

Today I mentor autistic people, especially young adults through the difficult years of puberty to mid-30's or even early 40's. I call these years 'the tunnel'. We journey these years in the dark, putting one foot in front of another not daring to hope for a good future. Every day is survival. That is why I have written this chapter. There is a way through a tunnel; it involves going forward. Tunnels are dark places, where a wider view is not possible. They are for going though and have a light at the other end. I am not the light, but I use experiences undertaken combined with skills gained to help the individual switch on their own light from within.

I like exploring old railway tunnels and I have these in mind when I came up with calling this difficult passage in life 'tunnel time'. On walking through a tunnel, the dark is something that no one on the surface can imagine; it is a complete absence of light. A soft, enveloping of dark that sharpens senses - navigation is by touch and sound only. One must reconfigure one's way of sensing the way forward. In the soft, damp quiet sound comes alive in a new way. It is a friend, the best sense one has of life and for sensing life. Breathing, heartbeats, clothes and soft measured footsteps are the soundscape. Damp, soot covered walls reflect no soft sound - they absorb echoes and give no sense of depth and distance.

The continuation of my own life is the sound that accompanies me. No distractions from sight, just sound, inner sounds and footsteps. That is like the intense inner life lived by autistic people in the tunnel part of life. Anything external is sensed with fear, incomprehension and sensory overload. The inner world is the one of life, the continuous one that counts the soft marking of time and life. Time in the tunnel is sensed softly and with a sense of mourning for the life that could be lived is we knew how.

Anger stalks us in this soft mournful world. People criticize us for... something we do not comprehend. Words of criticism surround us. Words of concern hurt our hearts. We do not know how to understand or respond, and days are lived in rhythmic steps, slowly padded to attract as little pain as possible. Deep nihilistic anger stalks and overwhelms at times. Suicide creeps along with the anger, offering pain relief and cessation of the painful journey without hope, or comfort. One step at a time, that's all; keep moving from darkness into darkness.

In that tunnel there is often a kindred spirit to walk with us. The kindred spirit must be sensed in the soft dark, but are often missed though sorrow and incomprehension. Occasionally, separated souls find each other and walk together. There are many mothers in the tunnel, looking for their autistic children, trying hard to understand their child's walk. Mothers armed with what understanding of autism they have, that has been written by non-autistic authors, so keep the instincts completely misinformed. But they do their best with what they have, often losing touch with their children in the soft incomprehensible dark to re-find them on hearing their screams of pain, when the nihilistic anger seizes their child. The journey is done in the dark and, more often than not, without hope.

Fathers rarely walk the tunnel. Often they are at the entry portal at a distance, willing protection on the mother and child inside to listen for them on their exit on the other side. Sometimes they hear the mother weeping when the child is lost, but she will refuse to come out and leave the child inside.

I have travelled the tunnel and came out into the light. Try walking a tunnel for yourself this weekend and on leaving the exit portal, notice how light and colours take on a new life, depth and vibrancy. The world is laid out in a vista like nothing that could be perceived without having gone first into the dark. Life is new and strong when back out in the light. Time in the tunnel has caused strength, perseverance, wisdom and a strong take on life that cannot be put out when back in the sweet light.

Much of my work is setting off back into the tunnel, carrying information and hope to the tunnel walkers. The souls carrying on in the dark, walking on alone, as that is all they can do. I set off back into the dark, carrying an eclectic mix of things - hope, pictures of the life ahead for the tunnel walkers, ways mothers can love, ways their children can know that love, giving permission to use stim objects and do whatever is necessary to keep their senses, mind and soul together. I walk a while with the mothers, help them see their child in the dark, understand their child and connect. Little things are needed, the right little things.

The autistic mind processes and seeks to understand all the time. The little things are the pins and turning points needed to make sense of life and grow hope for the future. We need to know that we can make connections in the tunnel and seek out friendships in the dark.

I tell stories of life in the light and help people prepare for it. Help them have faith in their own senses and plans for the future by giving little projects they can work on to occupy their minds and build. Ways to practice for life in the light, ways to prepare and how to think and learn their feelings so they can be ready. Help for the mothers to know they are good mothers and to have hope for their future too. No one is given a manual for their child and information is often so way off the mark when your child is different. Sense your child and travel with them. They need your love, even if they cannot communicate their love back for decades, it is there and alive. Love and hope are good for keeping anger and suicide at bay in the dark. For us autistics, information is useful to work out how to proceed and keep hope alive.

On my way back down the tunnel there are those who have fallen, having lost hope in the dark. They ended their pain. Their mothers walk on alone, clutching memories and what might have been. I feel unequal to the task of giving hope to the tunnel people. I do what I can with my stories, lights, explanations and guide ropes.

Sometimes there is a stationary soul unable to move on. Their energy spent and hope used up. That is time for a hope transfusion. I do not do many of these, as they drain all my energy and need long recovery times, but they are needed when all hope is gone. I leave the tunnel afterwards, sit in the clear sunshine and rebuild strength before going back in.

My wife and son are tunnel walkers too. We do our best to keep his hope alive, show him shafts of light, give him rest and help him on his way.

There are a few fathers in the tunnel, walking, feeling awkward and doing their best. Like most men, they do not ask for directions and bravely keep on course with their child in sight.

The parents crouching beside their motionless child, neither knowing the way forward having lost hope and strength, there on the floor waiting for... what they do not know and do not expect and have lost hope of finding.

The tunnel is large and can be seen everywhere when one knows what to look for. The girl quietly playing dead all her life, hoping not to feel too much pain. The young man, walking home with head bowed, hoping the bullies do not find him. The bedroom people who are not seen in public, living their tunnel time in quiet pain, longing for friends, the thin, young woman with no accurate body image, not daring to eat. The people in life's shadows, longing for friends and love, fearing contact in case they do not know what to do. The light of life all round them, yet not penetrating their darkness, incomprehensible in their sensory overload and fear. They must keep living, keep moving... to where? They hope a little, but do not know where to go. In life, and somehow not sharing it, while longing to live to the full, keeping on because they must.

They carry large weights of criticism, misdiagnosis, and hurt after failing so many times because they knew not what to do, sent quietly into despair by being defined as problems and negative ways of understanding their autistic lives. They carry all this pain close, lest they be criticised further for stumbling, or showing their pain, or slowing up because of the weight they must carry, keeping on because it's better than dying.

I know my life is to stay with the tunnel people being logically positive, useful and guiding them on into the light.

Keep True To The Dreams of Youth (Friedrich von Schiller)

The dreams of youth are the best and the purest forms of a person's inner life - where peace is found. I recall my childhood dreams and feel a deep inner happiness. Most of the time I cannot put these dreams into words; they are inner desires, feelings and a growing towards happiness and being really free in many ways of healing people. They are the peace I had when reading my Thomas the Tank Engine books. In those books, I entered a life of purpose and travel; a simplicity and a world I wanted to live in. In those books, people did things for the best, the engines were useful and the scenery clear and free, just like being on holiday in the countryside.

Useful - I wanted to be useful and have a place of value in the world like the engines. I wanted people to say I was useful and to want me. I wanted to be useful and be good at something, to be thanked and loved, to have friends and to feel secure in relationships with people. I wanted to have purpose and movement in my life, with people watching me go saying I was useful and good. I dreamed of all the things I could be good at. Nothing specific, but a common theme was being able to help people connect, light up and find what they were good at.

I remember hearing adults saying that they had not achieved what they wanted in life. If only they could have been a... with more money and they would be happy. I had no idea about jobs careers and qualifications, but I did know that people who liked what they did in life were happier than the others. I could not make out the connections and routes people took in life and how I would get to happiness and to be useful. It took me until my forties to figure this out. I wanted to be useful and for people to like me.

My young life was filled with disappointment, criticism and being called among other things - useless. I had a strong sense that people did not like me and my parents found me confusing, frustrating and a disappointment. I do not recall them expressing confidence in me. They expressed concerns. They pointed out my weakness and what I was always doing wrong. At school the teachers and bullies did the same for my confidence and self-esteem. As I grew, I became more painfully aware of the chasms developing between me and people. This process was beyond my comprehension and control, yet to my dismay and sadness, utterly discernable. All I ever wanted was to be useful and for people to smile at me and say they liked me.

Kick Back And Be Autistic

I've been mentoring lots lately and doing autism training for two other businesses I work for. I have also has three consecutive Sundays when I have been leading Church Worship.

Today is Sunday. I led worship this morning, cooked the Sunday roast, took the dog out and did the laundry. On Saturday, I was at a local event promoting my autism business, Autism Live Training which was very tiring - talking to people all day at a crowded venue with artificial lighting. I needed to script and re script all day long. Result - my brain is fried right now.

It's funny, but when selling an autism service, the last thing I can be is be true to my autistic nature. I've got to be very neuro typical in appearance and speech. A day of acting is hard work. I hear from actors that King Lear is a tough part for the leading actor, as his character is on in nearly every scene; they have no time to rest from acting during the play. When one is autistic one needs to act all day long.

Strangely a painful encounter was with an undiagnosed autistic man. He was about fifty years old and totally taken with cycling in our town. My public stall has a bicycle on it and he asked about the bicycle. Nothing unusual in that - lots of people do. But with this man, every question I answered led to another quick fire question, asked with more passion than the last one. He told me with conviction about the ideas he had for local cycling facilities. If I had any sense of self-preservation, I should not have mentioned that I am a member of the local cycle campaign group. Well... I did, and at this point he went off into hyper-autistic passion mode. He wanted to know so much about the local cycling scene and who was involved. He showed signs of an obsessive-compulsive personality and no awareness of the affect he was having on me, and how upset I was becoming. He repeatedly wanted to know the email of someone to contact about local cycling. I would not give him anyone's email addresses in order to protect the people I know.

Part of my stand included a laptop computer. I thought I would quickly show him the relevant websites, so he can pursue his interests and for my health leave me alone. That did not work; he just wanted to know more. I remembered the scene in *Uncle Buck* where Miles (Macaulay Culkin) asks consecutive questions to his uncle Buck (John Candy) until his uncle can take no more. When asked about asking consecutive questions, Miles answers 'I'm a kid, that's my job'. The man I was dealing with had not got the awareness that he was going too far in his probing and what is appropriate. Inside, my head was packing up and heading for a meltdown. Eventually someone else came to my stall and the man could not cope with two people and left. He took the wind right out of me; I was flattened and in severe overload pain. I stumbled on and spoke to a couple of people and then completely collapsed inside.

To regroup with my peace, I left my stall and went into church for a quiet moment. That moment lasted for over an hour – breathing and being calm in the quiet. After that time I had the strength to go back to the show and stay until the end, but I never quite recovered for the rest of the day. Once home, I reflected on the irony that the person who hurt me so much was autistic! However, there are some people who just can't read another person and let their interest become so overwhelming that people get overloaded with being kind.

I kept things together long enough to get through the night and be out again the following morning to take the service, but was not in a good state for a Sunday morning. I prepared as much as I could and stepped out in front of the congregation to lead the worship just as I have many times before. Then, being weary already, I was suddenly hit by the amplifier hiss from the PA system and my ragged senses were in such pain from processing this hiss that I visibly winced. When feeling prepared, I can normally work with interruptions and listen through the pain but I was so distressed and fragmented that I do not think I did very well at all that morning. It takes me about three days of peace to get over a severe and painful overload experience from another human being.

Anyhow, I struggled through the service and I stayed on my feet to walk the dog - dogs are nice, they don't chatter on like people do. I cooked the Sunday roast, took in the washing and was preparing my mind to do some work on the computer (correspondence etc.) with a cup of tea in hand. As I headed for the stairs, I noticed the television had been left on, showing a film *Batteries Not Included*, a film I had not seen since the 80s and one I recall enjoying. I was instantly sidetracked from the planned day. My wife was in the front room with a friend and I had the back of the house to myself. I felt elated - I could be on my own and watch a film I liked. I was in a reverie of being in the quiet with the film, a mug of tea and a comfy sofa.

I got utterly lost in the film, which is something I do not always do as I am usually active and restless. My senses were soothed and I felt my brain coming back on stream, a growing sense of peace grew up inside me. I felt cosy and at peace, and I can even feel the serenity now. All my stress and pain melted away and I thought how lovely it is to kick back and just be autistic, non-verbal and completely lost in a world of tiny machines. These moments are rare but I had no further ability to act like a neuro typical person and no expectation from anyone that I would... ahh bliss!

I hoped my wife would stay in the lounge with her friend for the duration of the film - if she came in she would want to talk to me and need my attention. I was healing at the time and could not handle a human interaction, since it was something I had just put a lot of effort into. I was mending myself, like when someone has an injury and finds peace in being still to heal. A difficulty for autistic people is when we take time to heal, people ask us what is happening - why aren't we talking or acknowledging them, why are we being antisocial etc. They just don't get it when we are deep in a reverie, building up resources for the next round of interactions where no one will let us be true to our autistic natures. That is like poking a physical injury and asking the person why they are so still and not moving normally.

When someone is physically injured there are outward signs of injury and people's stillness and quietness is respected. Who would think that poking a wound would heal someone or make them better? But with autism, poking our injuries with words and persistent interaction is normal. When we wince and show signs of pain we are criticised.

The film was bliss for over an hour, then my wife's friend left and she came in to see me. That is fine - I love my wife deeply and enjoy her company, but today she wanted to talk to me. I felt pain and was unable to respond, much like the same way a physically injured person does not feel inclined to move about much. Julie needed my energy and criticised me for being 'autistic' (something she says when she wants to talk and I don't). I tried to summon up the communication skills but couldn't manage many words - I just said 'I want to watch the film'. Just like my wife says when a programme she likes is on.

Unsurprisingly, my words were not well liked and she replied, 'So you don't want me with you?' It was not that at all. My soul was screaming out what I wanted to say from behind trapped doors marked sensory overload and she couldn't hear me. I simply had no reserves to draw on for interaction on a verbal level with anyone - I wanted to be my natural self - alongside her in the quiet and rest in her familiarity. She did become quiet after a while, but was not at ease with it.

I did get to finish the film. I did have to answer some questions and respond to some statements which caused distress, but not as many as I had feared. Being autistic I do like to have just one thing on my mind at a time, that day it was a film. I was away with the film, letting my brain get its act back together. Every comment or question caused pain in that it pulled me back from my introspection to think up an answer and how to say it, then say it and understand the follow up.

I managed to kick back and be autistic for a time. To have no other requirement on me than to be in the moment and be the autistic person I am does not happen much, and it's lovely when it does. Being autistic is fine in itself, and something I have come to appreciate, the peace to heal and just be true to my nature.

When I am being perfectly natural in my autistic way it must cause people to want to interact with me verbally. People appear to become more intent on verbal interaction. I wonder what signals they miss read. My best guess is that they see me at peace and assume I am ready for something, or that they see me so still they think it is a good time to ask me for something. Usually people ask me for something, or to do something for them when I am at peace and quiet. I don't mind being asked to interact, or do things for people, but I can't figure out why this happens most when I am kicking back, letting go and being my true autistic self.

Dear Susan – Letter To A Mother

I do feel for you. I have come across these situations many times. There is no easy way to deal with it. However, there are reasons autistic people lash out at loved ones. This often happens to people they love the most and who love them. An explanation of what is going on is rather like threading a needle with boxing gloves. But I will try…

The world of an autistic person is often a disjointed series of facts, events, feelings and frustrations. They can be systematised to some extent by the autistic person. But putting them into a cohesive whole can elude the person for years, decades even.

I will start with a Theory of Mind (TOM). This was first described by Permack and Woodruff in 1978. It involves 'the ability to impute mental states to oneself and others'. This is essential for human beings to be able to relate socially to each other and develop empathy for others. It is usually evident in children between the ages of two to three years. John will be developing TOM now. Autistic people have difficulty with this and may not develop a reliable and effective cognitive theory of mind for some time. Although we do read people, we do this with our autistic understanding, which does not help us interpret people's non-autistic ways. Some may only develop this deep into adulthood. To have a theory of mind, one needs a way of self-referencing one's own self, and to learn how to pick up on the many cues people give off as to their state of mind. This can be beyond the ability of many young autistic people, although it can be developed later in life.

Lots of parents of autistic children feel bad about the relationships they have with their children. They frequently say that their autistic child uses them and drains them of their capacity to emotionally connect with their child. This is a common occurrence and often down to the child not being able to reference their love for their parents and having little or no idea of the love the parent has for them. The child is often full of fear and on the edge of an explosive meltdown a lot of the time. The parent/child relationship can often proceed on a mechanistic basis for decades.

The autistic child does, in fact, love their parent and will have a strong sense of the parent's love for them. But, and it's a big but, they may not be able to effectively reference these emotions as a whole, so that they can make reference to and impute to the parent in their turn.

One counter-intuitive thing to typical people is the way lots of autistic people think (this is sometimes called Gestalt thinking). The world and people around them can be a series of unrelated facts. The person may not be able to make connections and form these into a cohesive model and comprehend the relationship between facts, life experiences, and crucially emotions. Autistics are gestalters - they make sense of things from the bottom up by assembling many details - until that process is complete they will not have an effective cognitive understanding of something. Love is in there somewhere but may not be recognised, linked to anything or be describable by an autistic person.

You will shortly see John form these connections together into a useable understanding and he will be able to show love back to you in new and beautiful ways, until he becomes a teenager. Teenagers go through final stages of neurological development before adulthood and for some years may have an impaired theory of mind. That is often why they become socially inept and can annoy the heck out of people around them. Autistic people develop differently in this respect and teenage years can be especially difficult.

John is unlikely to have developed much in terms of cognitive theory of mind yet. There are ways he can be helped to learn these skills. Often through systematic means - autistic people have a strong tendency toward systematic thought, as opposed to empathetic thought. They often have rather low 'emotional quotients'. This has become better understood in recent years.

I have not met John, so my explanation needs to be treated with some caution, but it goes like this - John's thinking contains many facts, feelings and life experiences. However, these are not very well integrated into a whole. Of particular difficulty and incomprehension will be emotion, especially love. It is there, but not well understood and could be frightening due to its strength. What emotion may be tangible is rage, fuelled by lifelong frustration and a lack of comprehension of life outside himself. This can be further fuelled by negative feedback from the non-autistic world through culture, misunderstanding, anger frustration and incomprehension of John's internal reality and his framework for viewing the world. This can form a Catch 22 throughout his life, generating anger and making self-esteem plummet.

John may also not have sufficient internal self-referencing ability to impute all this to his state of mind and how he interacts with other people. He will have even more difficulty recognising states of mind in people around him; this may be utterly incomprehensible to John right now. Because of this, he may not be able to understand that lashing out at someone and causing them a visible injury caused them pain, physical and emotional.

If he feels pain, he may struggle to reference it and work out where in his being it is located. Autistic people sometimes refer to themselves in the third person for this and related reasons. They may not have any self-image and refer to themselves as someone else, not their own self. They are frequently unable to feel their own existence.

Self-harm can be used to help get a sense of physicality. They feel they exist when they inflict pain on themselves. I do this several times a day but I have the skills to hide it so no one notices. This may seem counter intuitive, however it is a positive reason for self-harm in the perception of the person concerned. Self-harm also has another function; it causes the brain to release pain-killing chemicals like opiates. The self-harming person does it to feel better afterwards and as a means of destressing.

There is also a sense of pain on pain. Imagine someone is feeling chronic emotional hurt, punctuated by acute hurt as well. Imagine also they are frightened, cannot reference this or communicate it, due to being unable to reference it. Imagine the torment of carrying this through life as a hard truth that will not go away. Sometimes self-inflicted physical pain can ameliorate the other pain by providing a controllable dose of acute pain; the controllability of this pain being important to self-regulation. A sense of reference, purpose and comfort can be obtained.

This provides temporary relief from the chronic emotional pain, fear and self-loathing. This is the main reason why I insist that on my team, all autistic people are treated with unconditional positive regard. This can at first unleash a torrent of behaviours, noise and offloading. This is part of the autistic person resetting their emotional and self-esteem compass to a lovely place where we all like to be - happy, content, good relationships with ourselves and others and feeling fine. The process is hairy and it's a journey with a lovely end.

Things could be going more smoothly at Fielding House in part because the relationships John has with people there are not as emotionally charged as at home. There may be less to confuse John allowing him to comprehend the working relationship staff have with him. That working relationship is contractual, factual, professional, fostered and controlled in a working way. It may not challenge him as much as the deeper family ties. Also the absence of love in the mother and son relationship gives a simpler template for interacting with people.

I can recall many conversations I have had with parents when I used to run a respite care flat. So many mothers would feel bad at seeing their children doing well in respite care and said they felt that they were not doing well as parents. In fact they were wonderful parents and very good people who did wonderful things for their children. I always said that they are loving and caring for life 24/7 at home and with other family as well. At the place I worked, staff only needed to work for a few hours at a time then go home.

We could get nice long breaks that parents could not. The parents were in fact better at caring and bringing up their children than we were, they had more of it and were a lot more tired and stressed than us. Also, because it was our job we did, by necessity, work in structured and less emotionally involved ways than parents. This often suited autistic people who were finding close emotional ties and love hard to handle. We could always report in truth that the parents were loved by their children. The children had not yet developed the means to deal with this.

Decent professional involvement can be of great help in deepening – well, the depth of relationship is already there - rather oiling, facilitating and increasing the peace and flow of love in the relationship between John and Mum. There are many means of assisting John in his social and emotional development. It is not easy but it is possible. I have known many people do it. I get a lump in my throat when I recall families that were breaking down and filled with despair and self-loathing, turning around and growing close and showing love again. These times are highlights of my working life.

Autistic people are wonderful, fun, filled with love, integrity, truth, justice and a passion for life. We need help with self-esteem, making sense of it all, our place in life and family. I suppose the key to this is loosening up emotional reciprocity and the flow of love. I make this a cornerstone of any autism training I do.

Have a lovely Christmas all of you. And I sincerely hope your sister, John, and the children have a great life. They are in a good place for this to happen.

Richard Maguire

Autism Live Training

Living With A Matrix

In the autistic life nothing is random, half understood or done in a way that is disconnected from any other part of life. Life is a matrix of completely connected things on many connected timelines. I work with many autistic people and we have these frameworks for understanding and organising life.

Let's start from the beginning – for us, life as a baby is fine. Being held, sleeping in a cot and being adored works and we can feel good. Then we begin to move around, but we don't often crawl. Instead, we interact with the world according to our senses and understanding. People are an enigma, full of noises - they scare us or poke and prod us. As we turn into toddlers, they tell us off (don't do that, stop it you silly child and more negative admonishments) and we move through space as we sense it - unaware of our body size or the personal space and interactions that everyone else seems to do with ease. This is all a complete mystery to us and will remain a mystery if we cannot make sense of it. Most often we do not understand what people are doing around us, let alone be aware that rules to all this, with reasons attached that explain why they do what they do. It is all beyond our senses and comprehension. For us, people are often noises, shadows and morphing shapes. They are scary, not like the still objects in our homes which are often our friends and the first things we bond with.

Still, inanimate objects can be sensed and understood - emotions can be shared with them, unlike people who are noisy, touch us, move us and hurt us. We do not normally perceive faces, but are aware of the noisy parts of people in front of the hair. Hair is nice: it stays still, has form, can be stroked, is interesting and looks lovely in light. The noisy, moving part at the front is beyond understanding as its shape constantly changes - lots of pieces of it move and the noises it makes are startling. People around us expect that we should naturally appreciate the noisy space in front of the hair, but it upsets us, causes pain and is still wholly confusing. The shadows, movements and forces it belongs to hurt

161

us too - they move around our world, change colour, rearrange things that we found familiar and had made friends with and begun to orientate our worlds around.

The noisy thing is a face, the moving powerful thing is a body. The body appears in various clothes which is surprising to us, and we grow up nervous of people. As soon as we begin moving around and doing things, humans are the most frightening things in our lives - for me that has not changed. I am scared of people (even my own family). This is partly because I am conditioned to be frightened of people and partly because I cannot predict what people will do and say. I cannot do what people expect of me and the pressure is frightening and I feel horrid nearly every day.

I started at the beginning of this chapter to give an idea of how autistic child accepts life and what we are frightened of, spending a lot of time and effort dealing with the effects on us from interactions with people. There is nothing in the autistic life that needs fixing; as a system it all works well. However, we are a minority who sense, think and feel quite differently. This all adds up to a huge cultural difference between us and most people. And therein lies a difficulty - we are unable to conform to societal norms with any ease. We try hard to conform. I do not know how to express the gravity of how difficult this is and how much energy it requires. Even speech requires intense thinking and a concentrated effort.

Before I go on to describe the matrix, let's go back to the autistic way of understanding people and how we make sense of the world.

People are hard to sense and perceive because they give off too much information - especially the face, the blank incomprehensible area in front of the hair. Hair is okay as it just sits there and can be sensed. The face moves lots, noises come from it and eyes pierce our souls. Please feel free to look at details on our faces but eye contact hurts and frightens us. We do not interpret faces and the intentions of the person seeking eye contact. Instead, this information can be held for a long time unprocessed.

We feel the pressure to act, this causes anxiety, stimulates our limbic system and we immediately feel fear. It's the fear of being stared down upon by a predator. If you would keep your face still and avoid eye contact most of us would be able to recognise your face, remember it and be able to relate to you by your face. As this does not happen we normally go on your hair, especially its silhouette. On this point, if you change your hairstyle an autistic person will struggle to recognise you afterwards. This has caught me out a lot, especially with female colleagues. It takes me a while of checking clues like voice, movement and behaviour patterns to recognise someone I may know very well after they have a new hairstyle. Before reading on, please pause to understand what effect this has on our ability to socialise, get on at work, and deal with shop assistants, family or anyone else.

On top of this, people assume we have recognised them immediately. They think we need no time to process the many details they give off visually and verbally and that we can go straight into a conversation. If you are not autistic this may be possible, comfortable and even enjoyable, however, we are struggling to sense and recognise you. Our conversation will falter or fail to start and this happens every time we meet someone. It's a difficulty we have that goes unrecognised – often mistaken for rudeness. That assumption could not be further from the truth - we love people and desperately want to have contact, make friends and have a social life but struggle lots at having to do this in 'normal' culture.

We perceive many more times more sensory information than non-autistic people. Our senses are normally hypersensitive, meaning we are hyperaware. This is the sensory world of a nervous animal and that's a great analogy of what we are most of the time – alert, fearing predators with hyperaware senses. It is very tiring having to live constantly in this state, daily overloaded on adrenaline and exhausted - sometimes before breakfast. You, on the other hand, may be able to recognise faces and instinctively ascertain if someone is a friend or foe type personality. You can filter your sensory information and deal with only what you need to know but we don't have the brain structures to operate on an instant scale. Filtering and recognition systems are inbuilt into normal people but autistics have to take time to process the messages they are given – and feel the intense mental pressure of expectation as they do it.

That takes us back to our earliest experiences of dealing with people and the fear and incomprehension we carry from then on. Our lives start out in a raw sensory state - people have told us that we are wrong, naughty and being difficult. So we cannot live your way, but are unable to tell you that (as toddlers) except though 'challenging behaviours', and this state continues into adulthood. Instead, we learn quickly to act and behave in ways that are not natural to us. We are observers confused by your behaviours, yet at the same time we are trying to copy you, as this is the only way we are allowed to be and interact with people. Have a think about how hard that is. This state continues lifelong and we get tired very quickly - do you get this now?

We do not have permission from people around us to be who we are. It's a form of cultural intolerance combined with incomprehension. We do not live in the mainstream of human life and are unaware as children of how we and our behaviours are judged and viewed. We just know we get in trouble for being what we are. Then we must grow up, be educated and find work in this culture and struggle to be what we are not all the time.

We do know that we must get on with the majority of people and we are fine with that. Temple Grandin speaks plainly and clearly on our need to get on with people and for parents and educators not to let us tune out. There are many times each day when it is proper and legitimate for us to go the extra mile and relate to non-autistic people. However for us to be able to do this we need first to feel good about who we are, and have the inner strength to do this (difficult if lacking in self-esteem).

We autistics are treated in a negative way with regard to all that comes naturally to us. Furthermore, this is viewed as naughty behaviour, with the resulting negative effect weighing visibly on our self-belief and confidence. We begin to believe we are stupid and have very little strength to carry on. This negative model of understanding us is at the root of most of our failure to thrive and get on in life. I would suggest that anyone who is raised like this would struggle – and there is plenty of evidence in societies round the world to support this.

In my work I focus on two things first, one is helping the person find comfort in their life and understand who they are, the next is to find their natural means of communicating. The latter point becomes even more specific when the person has learning disabilities - they have to work even harder on communication. But, if one has the time to be still and take in their communication, they are gifted communicators. What they do is use a battery of communication styles and techniques.

They have not been able to master one technique because their neurology does not allow for this. Instead they use something called *total communication.* This is an eclectic style bringing in what they can do from verbal, gesture, object placement, their own placement, body posture, movement, sounds and anything else they can bring to bear in their communication. I have deep respect for anyone who communicates like this - it indicates a resourcefulness, holistic thinking and communication connectivity most of us do not use, because we have mastered one form enough to not need the others.

Most of us use speech backed up by body language and intonation. I do this too, as I am not naturally a verbal communicator - not many autistic people are. Autistics apply ourselves to learning and becoming proficient at whatever communication style the majority of people use, so I speak in English. However do not assume that because one of us uses speech that we understand speech to any great level. I don't, even though I have a huge vocabulary, which is all learned and repeated in something that is called *refined echolalia.* I am a visual thinker communicating visually with gestures and when with non-verbal learning disabled people I enjoy using this communication technique as it is my natural style.

I can hold a spoken conversation or one-to-one discussion on a subject I know quite well but if the subject changes or more people come in on the conversation, my auditory processing cannot handle and process the words. Speech becomes like the sound of shattering glass and I glean nothing. My son says speech becomes like the sound of running water when his auditory processing becomes overloaded. But in a lot of situations my son, many more autistic people and I pretend we are still in the conversation. We may go quiet or make verbal contributions that seem miss-timed and do not quite fit the conversation. What happens is that we fear social exclusion – I remember being told off for leaving a social situation and feeling gripped in a grim battle to stay there as long as I could.

I hope I have given you enough for you to have an understanding of some of our function abilities and how we seek to relate to people, make friends and get on in life. Now I can get on to the matrix as it serves a purpose in all this and is our means of placing ourselves in life - knowing how to deal with anxiety and get enough done before we melt down.

Given enough freedom to live the autistic life we would get on and go places in life with greater ease. However, we live in a world that is not set up for us to function naturally in. We are a minority. So we need a means of comprehending and navigating life - one built in to our cognitive and sensory world that enables us to interact outside of that. My term for this is to build a matrix of understandings to use for orientating ourselves in this foreign culture and navigate it with some success.

I will begin with sensing things. We autistics take in much more detailed information than most people. This is a fact, and we need to deal with it daily. We have our ways of handling this, but don't forget they take time and energy, which results in us becoming overcome with anxiety if we cannot use them. I recall Mark

Haddon talking on BBC Radio 4 about how he wrote Christopher's detailed description of Swindon Train Station. Mark said he spent three days in the station paying attention to every detail so he could write his autistic character's experience in the station properly. I recall Mark saying how tired he felt and how disorienting it was to perceive, remember and learn all these details.

It took Mark three days to pick up this information. It was information that an autistic person can pick up in a fraction of a second. Our feelings of disorientation and overload mirror Mark's closely. The research was done because he chose to so he could write Christopher's experience through the eyes of an autistic, and I think Mark shared these feelings with clarity considering most of the books giving insight into autism via fiction are written by non-autistics. Imagine a life where exactly that much information overload happens all the time everywhere? That's the autistic way of sensing the world. Do you understand now why we avoid things and places that seem fine to most people?

I remember driving home, after work, reflecting on Mark Haddon's words and the realisation took me - I really do take in the intricate level of detail more than most people. Mark gave me an understanding of the non-autistic life, where these inputs can be filtered and ignored so the main purpose of the day can be concentrated on and achieved, or switched on to be studied for fictional work over a period of measured time.

Autistics are very easily distracted by detail; we cannot filter them out and we will always sense them. To do this piece of writing, I am wearing headphones and listening to rain sounds to block out the auditory world around me. If I could hear it, I would not concentrate on writing. I would always have to know what the noise was and deal with it in my mind, which would mean no processing is left over for writing. Hearing is a pervasive sense and sounds travel - we cannot choose not to hear.

My sight is a little easier to deal with as light does not interfere with itself and travels in straight lines, so there are options like not looking or closing my eyelids. But to write I must see the keyboard and screen, so my eyes must be open. To cope with this, I arrange the screen in a set way to write and surround my computer with cameras to calm my peripheral vision.

Cameras are good for this as they are black, silver or grey. They are designed to be neutral, so they do not affect the colour of the light around the subject. A screen surrounded by these tones suits me as there are no colours to cause distraction. My arrangement of cameras changes day to day depending on the precise visual field I must have on that day. So here I am - rain sounds in my ears and soft greys and blacks around the screen. If anything is moved or changed by someone else I can no longer concentrate. When concentrating I must be on my own, as people provide too many distractions and these completely shut my processing down.

My computer is white, a deliberate choice, it does not distract me and I can comprehend the keys. The only colour near my computer is a blue and turquoise packet of Kleenex balsam tissues. I have a cold. I chose the tissue pack on colour only as turquoise is a relaxing colour for me.

The cameras to my left are, in front, an Olympus OM-2 with 35/2.8 Zuiko lens, and behind it is a Zorki 4K with a black Jupiter 8 lens. Behind these is a brushed silver card reader. I keep the card reader's cable unplugged and out of sight down the back of the desk, as it is too much of a visual distraction. On the right there is a brushed silver radio. Next to the tissue pack, in front of the radio, there are two cameras, and Olympus MJU-1 and a MJU-2, both piano black with rounded silver buttons on them and sculpted smooth forms. On top of the radio is a Contax T2 in plain unpainted titanium, grey and an Olympus XA, black, rounded with a red shutter button. I taste colours and a small red thing is a strawberry sweet. My memory stick, plugged into the side of the computer, is stainless steel and rounded in form so no distractions there either. All this arrangement around the computer is part of my matrix for concentrating and writing, change it and I do not write.

The matrix is a finely made web of connections that allow me to place myself in the world and interact with it. The matrix needs time and effort to maintain and hours of preparation to keep relevant and functioning.

If one part of a matrix is changed the whole matrix needs to be re learned and configured. Autistic people are very easily distracted and upset by sudden detail changes. We rely on our matrixes to keep our sense in order and make sense of the world. I often say in my training 'if you change one thing you change everything' in an autistic person's life.

Autistics don't start with concepts, we are bottom up thinkers and we start with details, then build concepts form these. If a detail is changed, it's analogous to changing one number in a spreadsheet - everything from there on is changed because of the changed number.

Another analogy for a matrix I use is the bicycle wheel. A bicycle wheel is round and its hub and rim are in the right relationship because of many spokes being in tension in a specific pattern. If the tension on even one spoke is altered the wheel will go out of shape. More serious than the initial misshape are the unseen tensions and misrouting of forces within the wheel. These uneven tensions will quickly make the wheel weak and will over-stress other spokes. The result first is imperceptible, but it will become apparent when the wheel fails completely.

To reach complete failure of the wheel may take months, but the process is in progress as soon as one spoke goes out of the correct tension. The fault is in there before it becomes apparent or seems serious. Being a cyclist and wheel builder I am quickly aware if spokes go out of tension, because I am aware of what is going on and can pick up on the first signs. Imagine someone is not aware there is a fault developing in a wheel; they could ride for a long time before there is a catastrophic failure of the whole wheel from what was originally a small fault that seemed trivial. I have seen bicycle wheels fail catastrophically and the result is painful and frightening. If maintained, a bicycle wheel is strong and will work for a long time without trouble.

The autistic life is like a bicycle wheel - a matrix of finely tuned things we arrange to help us keep on with life. We can seem to deal with one thing going out of tune without difficulty. We get criticized for spotting and raising the detailed faults in out matrixes. We are often told we are being fussy, not to mind and it will be all right. The trouble is that with the first detail going out of alignment our whole means of getting on with life is undermined, like the wheel. We can go on for a long time before things break down completely.

Like a wheel we will redistribute forces and explore all options for keeping things going. Most people do not notice this process, or the thing that started it. Most people are not autistic and do not need a matrix like we do; broader concepts and understandings will suffice. Being autistic and doing the work I do, I can spot these faults in the detail. From an autistic point of view there is no functional or emotional difference between a big or little issue. Intellectually we can explain the relative importance of things; this by the way puts a lot of people off the scent when working with us. They do not reconcile our factual intellectual explanations with the seriousness of details that seem inconsequential to them. They may think these details do not require attention.

I have seen a lot of autism work go wrong when this factor is not understood and the details are not given enough importance. Unknown to the non-autistic person, the whole process is becoming unravelled. The autistic person won't say most of the time. We fear people's reactions; they say we are being difficult, picky, fussy or worse. We get admonished and told to carry on as 'it won't matter'. When, in fact, something important has been left unaddressed, we will try and carry on. Because we do this, people become even surer these details don't matter. In fact, we are under a lot of pressure and very anxious. A meltdown is coming - its cause lay in the detail that was not addressed. The meltdown will occur when we have used up all our energy trying to cope with the situation and hold on to anxiety.

People have thought me strange when I tell them about this process and how important details and building detailed matrixes are. This normally needs some explaining, as does the idea that this is not about being fussy or difficult. It is fundamental to the way a monotropic, detail-focused thinker will deal with life. I teach people not to fuss or argue over the details, just accept them without comment. The comment will have to be put into the matrix by using a detailed understanding of it and its place in whatever was going on.

Often the less said, the better. That way an autistic person can build their matrix and proceed with life. When things need to be communicated, keep them detailed, calm and without value judgements or anything vague - that way they can be slipped into a matrix with maximum comfort and effectiveness. We can become overloaded particularly with verbal communication. When this happens it's time for quiet to allow for processing.

My life is one of simultaneously being hyperaware of everything and struggling to put this information overload into an overall understanding and plan for action. In social situations I am painfully aware of what is going on and unable to sort the information into a whole.

When I do manage to string some information together, planning to act on it is a struggle, even impossible if the overload is too much or I am tired. A matrix helps in that I can have a mental template pre formed that I can fit information into and plan from there. It is not perfect, and I can get this wrong, but it is better than nothing. If I seem socially clumsy or my words seem abrupt or inappropriate that is normally due to me being unable to form my verbal expression very well; I am working on ill-fitting and unfinished templates a lot of the time. This is usually done when under pressure to perform socially and communicate verbally. Remember, I am not a verbal thinker. I think visually with associated feelings and sensory attachments. These have to be considered, interpreted and put into words. Matrixes and templates help lots with verbal communication in that I use pre-prepared sets of words for expression.

I have been asked if learning-disabled autistic people make and use matrixes. I have observed this technique in use by every learning-disabled autistic person I have known. What is significantly different is that a learning-disabled person will simplify a matrix according to their cognitive profile. I say profile, as learning disability is complex with diverse developmental, sensory and cognitive profiles.

For example - I was working with a learning-disabled autistic adult, who wanted to do two things in town. One was to go somewhere to see some birds, after which he wanted to buy a drink to have with his lunch. After saying he wanted to do these things he paused and were quiet for several minutes. Eventually he asked if he had enough time. I answered 'Yes', then outlined a plan: walk to the water where the birds are, see the birds, walk back up the high street, and go to the Pound Shop (where he knew he would get two drinks for a pound). He thought about the plan, asked more questions about the route and wanted further assurance he would have time.

In fact he had as much time as he wanted, but that is an open ended concept, difficult for any autistic person. We like set points to orientate ourselves by. When he had processed enough he indicated he was ready to go. We went out and along the road then he stopped. He looked anxious, held on to me and began sobbing. We stood quietly for some minutes. Quietly he asked me if he could have the drinks he planned to buy. I said yes. He was still anxious and we waited quietly a few more minutes. More words faltered out, 'I have got a drink in my lunch box', another wait, 'can I drink the other drinks?'

I said that was ok - they can have more than one drink at lunchtime. I was asked how this would work. I said he could put all three drinks in his lunch box and drink one at a time. He could have drinks later too, or take a drink home. In doing this I gave him concrete understandable options he could build into a matrix, after first giving him cognitive and emotional permission to make any decision he liked. I also gave him a matrix to set his decision in. He spent a few more minutes thinking, then indicated he was ready to go. He did everything he wanted to do and followed the plan we had made.

The thinking and matrix building time took time. His sobbing indicated the level of anxiety he felt. The matrix I helped him build helped lots with the anxiety. I was specific – I avoided vague reassurance or vague encouragement (neither work in autism). He had his own motivation and desires; none was needed from me. Autistic people are often misunderstood as having low motivation when in fact we often lack a plan to proceed and are almost paralyzed by anxiety.

My words were to give the person a plan. If you were to have seen us planning and thinking we would have been still like statues on the pavement. Nothing much would have appeared to be happening, where, in fact, everything that needed to happen did happen - in the autistic culture, ways of thinking, communicating, planning and coping with emotions. We stood still so we could communicate and have time to think. I had built a matrix too, in the same quiet times the person I was with used. My matrix had more cognitive components; it included the things the person wanted to do, the routes, times, every contingency I could think of on the whole of the route over the whole time. This required me to run a lot of film in my head, so I had a film for everything I could foresee.

When we stopped on the pavement, I had pre-prepared several films to cover various reasons for stopping and what he might want to stop for. I ran my films, while acting and speaking as required.

The person I was with appeared to plan verbally - he rehearsed everything he needed to do, plus his concerns, with strings of words. As we went along he was checking off each point in the process, all the way down through shorter routines to silence on return. We both played out our pre-prepared routines to the end, and then both needed quiet to plan for lunch. If the person I was with had not had assistance to prepare his matrix and have his concerns addressed factually, with time to process and plan, there would have had a meltdown which would have occurred on the pavement where we stopped.

I have seen people try to cajole autistic people onwards in a situation like this, with only one consequence... a meltdown. The reasons being that they had no time to plan and deal with their anxiety - they would also have had their dignity taken away in the process. These events are remembered, resulting in them being unwilling to go again and be less inclined to engage with people. That in turn would lead to loss of confidence, trust, communication, hope and self-esteem.

The person I have written about used to be classed as having challenging behaviour. He is, in fact, a friendly, reasonable and communicative person who is autistic and needs to make up matrixes for every day and everything they do. He is a monotropic, bottom up detailed thinker who needs to line up all the relevant details to form a concept and a plan for life, just like any autistic person.

A learning disability means the matrixes need to be simplified and concise; it's quicker and less work, although I still need a huge amount of details. I would recommend learning from learning-disabled people, they can teach you a lot about how to perceive just what matters and discard all that is unnecessary for living life. They must use their senses, intuition and cognitive powers well. They are uncannily accurate and knowing. I think their skill is in living life well and avoiding unnecessary complication that the rest of us can get caught up in. If you want to learn how to live life wisely, in deep truthful relationship with yourself and everyone else, spend time with learning-disabled people.

My matrixes are very complex - I have the experience to do this. It is a burden at times. Often I have wanted to simplify like other people can. For years, I have watched people in action; they seem to be able to act and change quickly, to be doing things without a full technical understanding. They seem to have powers of 'getting though without all the facts'. All the facts make my head hurt a lot of the time, but I must have them to act. Assembling and carrying these facts feels like maintaining and carrying a heavy load. I want to go free of this load when I get tired. I try and I stop straight away for lack of a plan or any understanding.

There are times I get low, knowing what an effort it is to maintain these matrixes. I cry sometimes at the never-ending, grinding effort. I cry when people criticise me for being slow and forgetful. They do not know how hard I have worked to get this far.

There are times when my brain just stops. It goes inert; thoughts stop. Without a matrix and the mental energy to run one, I can still give a passable impression of being conscious and able. I call this going into a backup mode. I learned when young that people would not tolerate me coming to a cognitive halt. I developed a way of staying on my feet, keeping my head up, eyes open while running on a basic automatic set of responses, responses only, no thought or initiative, simply a survival mode.

This survival mode is painful. I do it though fear of people around me and a need to be included and not ostracised. I learned very early that when I was tired and stopped through overload, people rejected me. They said I was unreliable, lazy, and stupid and lots of other negative things. That resulted in me being cut out of whatever was happening next and ultimately being rejected. A fellow student on the Isle of Wight camp with me during my college years said to a new friend of hers 'Oh that's Richard... no one bothers with him'. I died inside when she said that. I thought I was coping and able to hack it with people my age. I felt a deathly loneliness in that minibus back to college. We were only together because of the space enforced by the minibus, not because anyone wanted me there.

We were at an adventure park, that morning on the camp. I looked forward to going, thinking I had friends. I wanted to go with the gang, go on the rides and share laughs to feel human and normal and not a freak. I remember when we got off the bus feeling alone for the whole trip. They made it clear I was not wanted, and I can still feel the acute pain recalling this. They paid attention to me only once, when I misjudged a zip wire and fell in a muddy puddle, laughing at me and finding my difficulty amusing for a minute or two. It was pain like that which caused me to develop my automated continuation mode after a meltdown or overload. I could not bear the bullying if I showed that I had collapsed inside - at all costs never show the pain. That is why I can appear to keep going when suffering a living death inside and all my matrixes and cognitive maps are gone.

I have surprised people in later years when I felt I could say I was in meltdown but kept going. They did not know of my automatic mode of operation. When in this automatic mode my sense and sense of time change - like stepping though a looking glass into a parallel world. I feel unreal and disembodied, time slows down and the pain seems eternal. My senses go numb. I move my limbs in what feels like slow motion, I hear my speech, limited automatic messages, only responses nothing initiated by me. I want to curl up and die. I hate living in the automated looking glass world. Sometimes this has gone on all day, like being at work and hanging on in there until I can leave. I did that at work because of the trouble I would be in if I told anyone what was going on, yet it was work that overloaded me and ran out all my matrixes and mental energy.

I cannot tell anyone when I am running on automatic, as they would ask questions which I simply could not answer and that makes the pain worse, causing them to say they dislike my attitude. So I just cover up and exist in pain until I can be on my own. A top tip here is - if you are with anyone who is autistic and they appear to shut off, or normal behaviour is suspended for reasons you cannot fathom, just be quiet in their presence. Ask no questions and by offering yourself as a benign presence, simply be and do not speak or act. The autistic person you are with will eventually trust you with this response and be able to repair themselves from the inside. Don't try to intervene; that will drive them deeper into overload and the pain they feel will be horrid. Many meltdowns are caused by well-meant intervention though words and action. Simply be a benign presence. That is just the level of intervention needed. It's like soothing a frightened animal, they want you to be quiet and with them. A frightened human is a frightened animal after all.

Only when inner peace is regained and overload is overcome can someone have enough cognitive ability and energy to make new matrixes and get on with life again. That is what I did with the learning disabled person when we stood still together on the pavement. They showed me when they were ready to go again - crucially they felt happy with the result.

This is one of the best ways of preventing meltdowns, not any sort of behavioural or sensory intervention I see so often. In my work I train people to be still; that is very important. If you are a parent you can do so much good by simply being you and offering yourself as the ultimate benign presence to your hurting, overloaded and frightened child. You will help them more than you could know and that help will carry on for the rest of their life. They need to learn that another human can be approached for comfort – show don't tell.

We can make and use our matrixes if we have enough encouragement, mentoring, information, energy, rest and self-esteem. We need to be told of the many possibilities there are, these are logged and used throughout life. We can become our own wheel builders eventually, fitting and tensioning our own spokes in our matrixes. Being able to do this is a key element to our liberation, happiness and success in life.

How frightened we are - and it's you we are frightened of.

My Lovely Family

I have more to say about my family than words can tell. Without my fantastic wife Julie and my wonderful son Josh I would not be here – it really is as simple as that.

Years back, in the dark days, I never thought I would have a family. I did not even think this was possible. I thought I was a nothing, that no one would love me. I was convinced I had nothing to offer as a father. No woman would want me. And even as a child, I used to try to get used to having no future and no one to love. I dared not hope, and settled in for a life of nothing – wondering how I would exist, maybe a continuation of the grey other world I lived in would be okay and I could get used to it. The trick was not to hope; never hope. Hope would cause pain though raising expectations of love that would never be fulfilled. The pain would finish me.

I got through life on stepping-stones of cycling, photography, walking, nature and the seasons one day at a time. I travelled, worked and kept busy. Alcohol was a useful pain reliever and loud music helped me feel emotions in a raw state. Around this, life was grey and slow.

One evening, I was invited to church service where a young woman was playing the flute. I liked her style and how she put emotion into the music she played. We went to the pub afterwards and I managed to sit next to her… I really liked her. I wanted to know her a lot better. Next came several pints of Marston's Pedigree to sooth my nerves and help me with finding the right words to say. She left early and I was lost without her there.

Later on, I learned that she too was autistic and had given up hope of finding love. She had no idea I was interested in her! It took me a while to find out where she was and to ask her for a date. If you have read the earlier chapters on how to process thoughts, replay conversations and prepare mentally for my daily living, you will know exactly how much I liked this girl in order to summon the courage to ask her out.

She was so surprised! I think it took her a while to know I was not having her on. I remember that first evening in a local pub. She played the machines most of the time. I was happy to drink beer. Not many words passed between us. Two autistic people spending time together. That's more than OK.

We go to know each other better and it was not long before we were engaged. We married two years later and eventually our beautiful son arrived, who has exceeded even our wildest expectations.

I wondered if I could be a father. I knew so little and had no confidence in myself. When Joshua was born everything seemed so natural. He is fifteen now and doing very well. We are close like brothers, sharing the same silly sense of humour and interests.

Several times a year I visit somewhere we went when I was younger. I do this to take stock of life now and how good it is with my family – just the three of us. All this came when I was not looking or even hoping.

What would the ideal conditions be for parents completely failing to spot autism in their child? If both parents are autistic... as far as they are concerned their child is growing up normally. It was a teacher at secondary school who spotted Joshua's autism.

But You!

But you? I hear this lots said to me and other autistic people. I can talk, go out, do a job and appear quite non-autistic a lot of the time. Then people seem confused when something autistic becomes apparent. I appear not to be autistic because I run overlays of skills, routines, language, posture, stop stimming (stimulating repetition such as leg shaking or tapping fingers....) for a while and generally work hard at pretending to be what I am not. All of us 'autistics' (I hate the word sufferers) do this as is as much as we are able.

What confuses people with me, and others like me who can run a lot of overlays and routines that hide autism, is an expectation that I can do this all the time, or that I am not autistic at all. People express shock and surprise when my autism shows in an overt way. They often say unkind things such as 'don't be so rude' or 'pull yourself together' before saying nothing more or launching into a great deal of criticism. I often get excluded, bullied or sidelined from all manner of activities including work.

Once things go wrong in this way I cannot normally repair the situation or deal with the fall out and get back to a comfortable situation. This usually requires skills and quick thinking that are way beyond me at the time. If I could have two weeks to think and script responses that would be better, but how often does one get any time to think at all?

Life being autistic or different in any other way, I suppose, just cannot be easy nor lived on autopilot. Creativity, persistence and an ability to take pain go with having a different sort of life. The things that cause the autistic life lie hidden in our brain. The effects of this show in the ways we live. People seem to find the absence of an obvious physical difference hard to comprehend. They frame our behaviour, communication and sensory differences in terms of behavioural issues. We frequently get reproached for not trying hard enough or being ignorant. And it pains us to know we are being genuine - yet dig deep to smooth over and cover up for what we really are and act like something we are not. Acting is normally okay; we know the need to get on with people and to frame our lives in ways they can comprehend. However, it all gets too much when we must fend off criticism as well.

When with an autistic person you will perceive a lot of coping strategies. We would have to be very trusting or tired before we would show you our autism in the raw. Only learning-disabled autistic people will show their autism in the raw most of the time, more so if they are severely learning-disabled. Then you will see a real representation of what they are with little affect or pretence.

With me, you will see the product of coping strategies learned and developed over forty plus years. I do not have the ability to hide my autism all the time. When I cannot do this I will usually stay at home, upstairs in a room. At these times I am tired and do not have the strength to cover up and act. I do not go out at these times, if at all possible, as to interact socially is too much. I also know people are shocked, and I think they feel uncomfortable when I am autistic in the raw. They are used to the cover up me, not the real me.

When I am not covering up I am nonverbal, will stim and appear like a learning-disabled autistic person. I have been shown in no uncertain terms that people will not accept the uncovered me. They say I am getting worse or have become more autistic. They give negative value judgements, question my integrity and anything I might be doing that involves them. When I was a child I would just be attacked. I quickly learned to cover up when I went to school.

Imagine life spent pretending to be something you are not and acting in ways that run contrary to your neurology. Is that a life you would like to live? How much strength would you have for dealing with people and everyday tasks? How would you feel about yourself? How tired would you get? How anxious would you be? How much preparation would any social contact need?

After all of the above, add in criticism based on a misunderstanding of the cause of autism, in neurology. People will tend to understand autism with the frameworks they have for understanding behaviours. We don't look obviously different. It would take someone with an in depth knowledge of autistic people to spot the subtle motor, posture, facial and eye contact differences. If they do notice, most people do not have a framework for understanding this and we appear odd.

People with a deeper knowledge of autism can still criticise us and cause hurt. It's not deliberate in most cases, as there is still not an informed enough understanding of the autistic life, causing them to misunderstand us and comment with non-autistic neurology and life in mind. I see this in a lot of specialist services and schools - people have lots of knowledge, yet have not developed enough understanding of how autism works out in the lives of those living with it.

When training staff, I take them through exercises designed to experience the cognitive and emotional world of autism. They learn lots from this and my accounts of how the autistic life is lived. I frequently hear from the people I train that they understand autism differently and will work in a wholly different way when they return to work.

So if you are ever puzzled by the presentation of an autistic person, please don't use the words 'But you?' We have heard them a lot - usually as the beginning of an uncomfortable sentence, laden with misunderstanding and criticism. What you will see are two phenomena - one being the level of acting and autism covering ability someone can come up with, and two being something of the profile of someone's autism. What you see immediately will give no information on how autistic someone is. We are all autistic with different profiles and levels of anxiety affecting our coping skills at that moment. That's all; it's not about severity.

People

I have been writing for years and lately I asked myself - where have all the people gone? I could see few people in my writing, which is mainly situation and explanation. And, I wondered why they are not there and what I could write. I thought about this for a long time, thinking in turn of everyone I can recall. I can recall lots of memories about the people I have met. I have lived with people all my life, and relationships with them are central to my life, most of all my parents, sister, wife and son. How could I leave these people out? Yet they have very few mentions.

I went deeper into my mind, recalling people, and sought to make descriptions of how much I loved them, but both a lot and nothing came. Lots of information, in that I have many memories of people and experiences with them, but nothing that would add up to recount. What I can recall is clear, yet fragmented. I tried to put these fragments into whole pictures of people with little success. What I could get together got lost at translating them from visuals to words. Things just would not hold together long enough for me to grasp and translate shapes and sounds using my matrix of understanding.

So, how can I write these many clear yet fragmented thoughts down? I struggled with this and the more I thought the more clear fragments came making wholes out of them became harder. It is as if the thing I am pursuing is on the horizon, in sight and looking within reach. Then as I head for the horizon it recedes at the same rate I am going towards it. The thing on the horizon is equally out of reach, all the time. If I run the horizon runs, if I walk it walks, the horizon and I do not meet - all this clarity within stays out of reach.

Then I thought, that is what people are all the time... details out of reach. Even my family, who are so close to me, are something that I run after in my mind to understand, and that understanding runs of ahead of me. I have occasional moments when my family appear lucid and whole; I try to hold the moment as I do this, but the understandings I have are fragmented and trickle though my mind like glitter though my fingers. I feel frustrated and alone - they are so close, yet beyond me. I love them so much and still struggle to give this wholeness and live the moment with them.

People, to me, are like the night sky - a universe of countless stars, bright shining yet incomprehensible as a whole. I look at the stars in turn, and maybe a constellation if I can. Each one is whole and clear when gazed upon individually, but the whole night sky is beyond vision and comprehension. I look out at people - seeing them through a telescope, one telescope for each person.

Many telescopes I can look down on and in turn see something. In these telescopes, I see a detail, but not the whole person. I move the telescopes to scan people, their movements, moods and changes. Each one is spotted and logged, then they trickle away like a thousand sparkly things. Each sparkle was a clear detail that I could not put into a whole. The whole continues to elude me. I look around on the floor for the pieces of glitter, picking them up and hoping to get enough in my grasp to see a whole person. No matter how much I pick them up there are always pieces of glitter left, leaving the whole picture incomplete. I want to perceive and know people well, and perceive them clearly, and I grieve over the loss of information all the time.

I look at people, not too much so they don't get uncomfortable. I scan for details, seeking a whole. People move and change continually, so my details are always out of date and distorted through the movement, so, no, I have no big picture for anyone. I can perceive lots more than most people it would seem, maybe too much. My brain races to keep up dropping things on the way. I do have one chance and that is if people will be still for a while. I can drink in details and begin to see them as a whole.

I know more about my wife and son from when they are asleep. The visual memories I carry are more complete if they are peaceful within themselves, and sleeping is the best time to capture these precious moments. Moving faces and limbs, I struggle with, needing to be somewhere quiet to process what I know about my family that love me so much. I feel sad when I am away from them as I can remember very little about them, but there is something magical about seeing them for the first time each time I see them, and it makes my heart leap.

There will be very few people talked about in this book, although I know and am in deep gratitude to many. I simply cannot pull the information together to write about them. They are very important to me and frustratingly indescribable with words. But they know who they are and that is enough for me to thank them.

Photography

I have a small, square photograph taken in 1970. The people in the photograph are my mother, myself, my sister and my grandmother. We are sitting on a bench in a park. We had posed for a photograph and I remember my father standing tall - silhouetted against the clear blue sky. His elbows were out to the side as he held the camera. In the picture I am holding a camera to my eye, framing my father in its viewfinder. I wanted to take a picture, and I remember my father advising me not to. He said the picture would not work because of the bright sky behind him - light would leak round and obscure his image. He said there would be no detail in him. He went on to say that the lens in the camera I was holding was not good enough for the picture I wanted to take, and the lens in his camera was much better.

I wanted to try with his camera but my dad said that the camera he used was complicated and I would have to learn more to know how to use it. That was it; I was hooked on photography. In that short conversation I learned there was a lot more to photography than I could have guessed. I wanted to know what the differences were with the cameras, and how with the right camera I could get the picture. My mind reeled with the possibilities as I saw the whole world in pictures, and with the right camera I could record it. More than that I could engage with the world too - with a camera.

I used to look though viewfinders, imagining the lives and worlds that were framed in them. People I could not comprehend in real life became discernible and knowable though a viewfinder. For a few seconds, I had a deeper relationship with my father, found through the viewfinder, than I could recall. I kept picking up the camera to see people - hoping that that special few seconds of conversation, relationship and happiness could be repeated. I used to see my dad over his shoulder while he was driving, from the back seat, through the viewfinder. I tried to make conversation again, several times but it did not happen again like the first time - I did not understand this at four years old, wanting to constantly repeat the magic with the camera and feel happy again.

I suppose that is what I have been doing in the years since, looking into viewfinders wanting to connect and be happy. Even as an adult I can still see and perceive people much better though a viewfinder, in fact I can perceive anything better in a viewfinder. It's comfortable, precise, surrounded by black and peace. I can watch anything and anyone though a viewfinder. The viewfinder is my cognitive filter – it takes away the overload and places life in a beautiful pool of light and love, where I can connect.

Last Sunday it was Father's Day and we went to a pub for lunch. Seeing the world through autistic eyes with my back to people in the unframed world - Julie to my right and Joshua to my left - I felt happy. I took a photograph of Joshua while he was thinking. Up came the camera, and though the viewfinder I saw him clearly, my lovely son, moving, living and being himself. I was able to discern his mood, connect with that and take a photograph, which was my emotional connection with him. I have not had the film developed yet, but when it is I will have my dear son recorded, with all the emotions I felt in silver halide on a piece of cellulose, an image, memory and emotion to keep and cherish.

Julie, my wife, says that my photographs show emotions I do not display in the rest of life - they are full of feeling. The word display is right, I have emotions everywhere and for all of the time, but they are frightening and out of bounds for comprehension in the unframed life. Since that day in the park with my father, I got an idea of the potential of the camera and being able to record what I saw in the viewfinder for life. I wanted to take pictures every minute, of everyone I knew and met, of everywhere I went. I wanted a memory of photographs and to live the feelings that went with them. I can look at any photograph I took at any time and I am transported in my mind, straight back to the place I took the picture, reliving the feeling of what I felt then - recalling the thoughts clearly too. I have no other way of getting to feelings or people that is anywhere near as effective as with a camera.

Photography

Back home in the kitchen, in a drawer, was a Kodak Brownie 127 camera. I held it for hours and carried it around. It had a viewfinder, a little dark tunnel with a rectangle of clear light at the other end. I framed up everything I could with that camera. I used to click its shutter, take the back off and see its simple internal workings. I did not know what the film did when I was four, but I knew a camera had to have one to be complete and work. I remember Kodak films, red and yellow things around spools. I did not like the cartridge film our instamatic camera took, the camera that I held in the park - the film was just a black plastic thing with a small window showing the presence of red and yellow Kodak inside.

I remember going to visit a friend of my parents where their son, who was older than me, used and reloaded his camera. I remember him taking the back off and saying a new word 'exposed' and seeing the Kodak film being removed before another was carefully threaded in. I remember it had two lenses on the front – lovely, purple tinted pieces of round glass, like jewels. I wanted lenses like those. The ones in our Instamatic and Brownie were like frogspawn, small and clear, so I wanted to understand the difference. I heard my dad saying that the purple tinted lenses were 'coated' or 'bloomed' and, according to my dad, that was better. These types of lenses could deal with all sorts of light.

I learned that cameras with 'coated' lenses had something called 'exposure control'. Exposure control had something to do with the milled metal knobs on the cameras (the Instamatic and Brownie did not have the metal knobs and no exposure control). Exposure control sounded important; my dad and other men would look serious and drop their voices when talking about things like that in relation to cameras.

I knew the camera my dad used in the park had metal knobs and a pink lens, so it was something of very great interest. It contained mysteries and good things I wanted to explore. That camera belonged to my grandmother, and she did not like it. I was confused by her attitude to it. She said it was hard to work and made her fingers hurt on the stiff metal controls. She wished she had an Instamatic camera like my dad. So there was a mystery to solve here. Serious men liked the cameras with coated lenses and exposure control, whereas my grandmother and other women, including my mum, liked the plastic simple cameras that were easy to use. Different opinions, all sincerely held, by two groups of people. I felt like I thought the exposure control cameras would be better for me, but they hurt people's fingers - a puzzle I set out to solve.

In proper autistic style I held on to that puzzle, and even though it took me ages, did solve it. The answer is like this - the exposure control camera my grandmother did not like was something called an Agfa Super Isolette, with a fold out lens and rangefinder focusing. That meant the shutter and focus controls around the lens had to be made small to fit in the folded camera body. To get grip on them these controls are machined and milled from aluminium, small and stiff. Therefore they hurt the tips of people's fingers when using the camera. The controls allow access to a compur shutter, aperture blades and very accurate focusing, which are all important if precise control and accuracy is desired. That makes the camera stiff and slow to use, but the results are spot on if all this control is done properly.

However, the Instamatic is cheap, simple and not nearly so accurate - but it is optimised to make pleasing pictures under bright sunlight, like when on holiday, thus giving someone a choice between technical perfection and recording a holiday snapshot. People decide what their priority is and choose a camera accordingly. This differing of priorities helped me a lot in life. I learned young that there can reasonably be more than one view of something. That is something I teach to autistic adults, which is so important to learn. We can often get into trouble because we may not know how to hold a differing opinion based on different information and priorities from other people. Misunderstanding this can lead autistic people into difficulties - it's fine to have a different priority and do something different about it. I am pleased I learned that one young, really I am.

Photography

Today I read angry arguments on internet forums between autistic people interested in photography. One thread I read involved an argument over the resolving powers of various 35mm lenses and which is better. I was sad to see how nasty and personal people were getting. I have two of the lenses being discussed and yes they are very different in how they project images onto film. The explanation for the differences is simple: the designers had different priorities. So what? I have both, and I choose the lens that will help me make the images I want for different subjects.

The lower resolution lens helps make pictures with balance and subtlety, the higher resolution lens produces very finely detailed pictures. The resolving power of a lens is but one of its qualities to be held in balance with others. Sadly some, maybe quite a lot of, autistic people don't seem to grasp this idea that one does not need to chase absolutes in life. Fuzziness and nuanced judgements are very useful and help us feel happy with ourselves and other people of deferring views.

I do a lot of mentoring with adults, and it is essential they learn this. I wish to thank my mother, grandmother and father for helping me learn this though my interest in photography. I also wish to thank a family friend, Ken, for helping me with this. He used to work for Kodak and I listened to him talking about films, cameras and lenses. He spoke of optimisation of these things to enable photographers make pleasing images, absolute values he said would make very poor photographs, nothing in the process should be made to be absolutely something or another. It was better if they were all good, not perfect, that way they would all work together.

Ken's specialism was film; his camera was a Kodak Retina. He spoke of its limitations and how he needed to be creative to get round them to make good photographs.

From Ken I learned that imperfection and limitations caused us to be creative and feel our way into what we like doing. Again, another powerful and useful lesson was learned. I carry that lesson on into my adult life too. Don't do myself in trying to achieve technical perfection. That is something I reach when mentoring autistic people too. Every time I lift a camera to my eye these lessons and a lot of memories come flooding back.

Lifting a camera helps me to orientate myself in life. A top tip I give is for autistic people, and some non-autistic people, to have a talisman like this to help them ground and reorient. I will hold a camera for a time when thinking and feeling, that helps a lot. I feel calmer and have a better idea of how to proceed.

My other grandmother used to work in a chemist where they handled photo processing. I got a lot of wisdom via her and recall taking the Instamatic camera on a day out to a museum. I took photographs of steam engines; while doing this I saw their shapes and forms, wanting to experiment with perspectives and vanishing points. In the viewfinder I saw beautiful and fun ways to frame pictures. Later, back at the chemist shop I heard most of my pictures did not come out. My grandmother's colleague said I needed to use a different camera to get the pictures I wanted. The Instamatic was too simple and did not offer enough control to get the focus and exposure right for these pictures. I was off again on an autistic mission to understand why!

I remember seeing an advertisement for a camera system: Nikon 'The Camera Never Lies but the Lens Can Bend the Truth'. The advertisement showed pictures taken on various lenses showing how the lenses could represent reality differently. I was looking and learning, lenses, viewpoints, exposure control it's coming together.

Once, when we were out having a family drink at our local pub, my dad had his camera with him. It was a Zeiss Ikon Contarex - big and shiny with changeable lenses, dials and controls. I wanted to take a picture. Dad showed me the meter and controls and I can remember that exact moment when it all fell into place: how to make a photograph while being in control of every part of the process. It was very exciting to know that with the right knowledge I could take a photograph of anything. I was allowed to take a picture, my first venture into making a photograph while knowing exactly what to do and why. I photographed a horse in the field at the back of the pub. I focused, metered and compensated for contrast in the scene so the horse would come out just right.

The film was Kodachrome, a slide film that needed very precise exposure. I got it right first time. I still have that slide somewhere; it comes to light now and then. Making that photograph was a pivotal moment. I had mastered something that gives me a lot of happiness, allows me to see, frame and give emotions expression. To make what I see in the viewfinder a recordable reality every time, everywhere. I went around framing photographs in my mind's eye then. Using the Contarex in my imagination, I could conjure up every visual, tactile and auditory part of the experience.

I could not afford film, but the joy of knowing what to do was complete. I still feel that joy now and recall that day every time I take a photograph, that day I cracked it. Years later, I worked over the summer in a cycle shop and earned enough money to buy a camera with full exposure control and a good lens, something I could use to give full expression to photography. I still have that camera, a Pentax K1000. It cost one hundred pounds and three pence from Dollonds Photographic in Aylesbury. Link anything to a camera or photograph and I have total memory recall.

Top tip – link-learn development and experiences in the autistic life to real things, our passionate interests. We will learn and remember – that's how our brains work. Always avoid generalities and vague concepts with us we will not get cognitive purchase on them and will stress out over what we should know and don't know. We also need good, precise advice and mentoring. We can go and make mistakes and repeat them due to a lack of quality accurate specific information. Remember we don't do vagueness or unrelated concepts.

We get concepts when we have enough information to build a concept - first we need good factual information and lots of it, so we can model concepts and see the bigger picture. I got good information about which camera to buy from a professional photographer, Tim Hughes. I told him I had saved up for a camera and wanted to know what he would recommend. He gave me new information to consider and explained lens quality mattered most, then good build quality, reliability and good ergonomics. Brand new information here - lenses are not all equal, not even the metal bodied coated lenses. He recommended two cameras with good lenses and good handling within my budget. One was the Olympus Trip, an automatic camera with a good lens and build quality. The other, more expensive, the Pentax K1000, I gulped at the price. Tim reassured me that if I could afford it the K1000 would be a basis for my hobby to grow and to have complete creative control over taking photographs. With that information I went for the K1000 and never regretted it.

Another top tip - when advising or mentoring an autistic person, give the best quality information you can as they will make firm plans and ideas based on that information. To make corrections later on is hard. If you do not have the information, refer the autistic person on to someone who has. The information will be used well.

My visual mind had taken in photographs from other photographers too. My mind seems to have a limitless capacity for images; I have to be careful, though. I can get so into images that I forget everything else in life. Tip - don't let an autistic person tune out everything that is not within their special interests as they will miss so much of life if they do this. There are times when I will deliberately not take a photograph; this discipline helps me stay tuned in to everything else.

I am never far away from a camera, loaded and working, although I will go out without one sometimes. Over the years I have marked life events and stages in life thought the pictures I took and cameras I carried. On occasions, I revisit old subjects with the cameras I had at the time. I did this today before writing. On my morning dog walk today, I took an old Pentax and photographed some subjects in ways I did over 20 years ago, with the same camera and lens combination. This allowed me to take stock of life, how far I had come and how to love life today and live well, loving my family and tending my enthusiasm for life.

The photographs I made will go down as way markers, memory makers and prompts for the future. The process of making photographs all links in too. Holding and using a camera and getting my body into the right position pulls my senses, mind and body together. I live in the moment the picture is being made, and live in the process. I balance my body, getting a sense of where it is and how I am holding it. I hold and turn the camera's controls, getting sensory feedback from hands that are normally remote and do not feel like they belong to me.

In the viewfinder, a piece of the world is described and comes into focus. At that time, life, the world, my senses, mind and body come together and it feels great. I planned in my head everything I would write today - in those moments behind my camera. If I need any prompting or recall I just go back to the images in my head and everything else comes back to me in harmony. Later there will be photographs too.

August 1988 was a time in life marked by photography. I had been through my worst times, depressed, suicidal, breakdowns and in August I was restarting my life. I was unemployed for six weeks, then I got a temporary job in a factory and that felt good. This was my last day before starting the job. I went to Oxford to wander around the colleges and by the river, looking at the light.

I also like, and still like, the bicycles parked everywhere. I get lost in their forms and colours feeling deep relaxation and happiness. Back then, Oxford had several photographic shops which I would visit in turn. My favourites were McNeil's in Turl Street and Jessops in Queen Street. For a while I had been interested in a camera called a Pentax P30n. It would complement my Pentax K1000 by adding another body with automatic exposure, as well as the manual I was used too. I liked its look, handling and clean appearance.

I checked the shops and Jessops had a P30n with a lens. I did something I would not normally have done and bought the camera on an emotion. It felt great. I soon had it loaded up and going. I remember that walk from Queen Street to The Pain, just beyond Magdalene Bridge. Today 25 years on, I can recall the entire walk, including views through the viewfinder – because that purchase was at a time of a new start in my life.

I had the P30n for a number of years and loved using it. I took it to Iona Abbey at Easter 1990. A group trip to the abbey had been organised by my local church. One of them, Donna, was a colleague, and she told me there was a space left. I got it. That Easter was the confirmation of the turning point that began in late 1988. Those days at the abbey changed everyone who was there. I remember people from all over the world in pilgrimage to the abbey. People of many cultures and languages all gathered in Christ. We all accepted and loved each other as we were. I do not know how to express by any means how important that was. My life had been mostly failure and rejection because I was different, but there, in the abbey, I felt interesting and likeable.

The Pentax P30n was with me all the time. I took black and white pictures with it, a new exploration of light, life and people. I have all those pictures. Two are on Flickr (Richard Maguire cycle.nut66) at http://bit.ly/14IdfGl for a picture taken in the cloister and http://bit.ly/13h2RcM for one of the first pictures I took of people. I remember taking these pictures as if it were only this morning. I marked and celebrated these moves in my life the way I know how, with photographs. For the first time I had such a good connection with people – I could ask them to pose for a photograph and we all enjoyed it.

From those ten days in 1990, I began photographing more people, because I connected with more people and had found a way to take their pictures. People mean more to me than things, they always have. It's just that I had not the means to connect with them when I was young. On that day on Iona I knew I had several friends. That was the beginning of my new life - all felt and documented though photography. Like my wife says, my emotions show in my photographs. Please do take a look at the shots by clicking on the link (print costs mean I cannot show them here).

I traded that P30n in on another camera a long time ago. I miss it lots, it held so many memories and helped me to make them. Years later I bought a Pentax P30t a successor model, only changed a little from the P30n. The associations are so strong that when I use my new camera I can literally see those views from 1988 to 1990 in its viewfinder, if I want to. I can even overlay two images in a viewfinder and play them like videos. In a viewfinder my life, feelings, thoughts, history, and memories can come together. In all this, that P30n carries the most hopeful and formative memories, I frequently take stock of life and use the memory of that camera to hold them all together.

Since I parted with and missed the P30n, I have not parted with another camera if it has deep memories and emotions attached. I cannot get that camera back as I have no way knowing which one it is. Today the P30t and the photographs from back then are good enough.

You may have discovered, from reading my scribbling here, that autistic people will form bonds with objects before and with greater ease than bonding with people. This is true in a lot of lives. An object stays what it is, it will not overload us, and we can keep track of it and refer to it any time. We will bond with objects often, not because we prefer them to people, but because we must. People are beyond our reach in sensory terms. That puts people beyond our reach in emotions and love also. I recall grieving over lost love with and from people as a child. I longed to be close to them and feel properly human in relationship with them. But I could not, so objects had to do, the first ones being soft toys.

A lot of autistic people will carry an object, and mine is a camera. These objects fulfil a need for connection and comfort in a world that is normally beyond our senses, emotions and grasp. We would rather make connections like we see other people do, but these elude us.

I shoot film, lots of film. Subtlety, life, tone and everything visual comes together on film well. I do have some digital cameras and use them, but, oh dear, digital is so clunky and unsubtle compared to film. It's deep, technical and down to properties of both photographic systems and boils down to this - digital sensors use millions of photo sensitive cells arranged in a grid to sense light and make electrical signals. These signals are translated into digital values, from which a file is made that can be opened by a computer to show a photographic image and printed when required.

This system is much less subtle and sensitive than film, the sensor cannot resolve any detail smaller than it's uniformly sized light sensors, nothing bigger either. That makes digital sensors incapable of resolving very fine detail and recording the subtle detail and tonal details in life. Maths is used in digital photography to give the impression of fine detail and subtle tonal gradations that the sensor could not detect. Film on the other hand records tone and details naturally in one go at the time of exposure, nothing else is needed. Film will record detail and tones that a sensor cannot, giving film images a feel and life digital cannot record, and it does this naturally with no further interpretation.

Film helps me think and connect life and senses. Film needs to be got right straight away when the exposure is made - you don't 'Photoshop' film. A film image is made with care, it cannot be erased, it must be right. A film image cannot be checked straight after exposure. A film photographer needs to be sure enough of their photographic skills and way of seeing the world to know the picture is right the instant before it is made. That requires a deep sensing of the world and knowledge of one's relationship to the subject. That requires connection and insight. I need that connection to connect with life.

If you can, have a go at making photographs on an old, metal-bodied manual film camera like the K1000 I bought. Every stage of the process requires the photographer to turn metal controls, which are mechanically linked to the cameras inner workings. You must make every decision, and the camera will faithfully carry them out for you. Eventually this process becomes intuitive like any skill that is practiced over and over. It is possible to take better pictures, faster and with an almost 100 per cent success rate on a manual camera. Then there is the satisfaction, when seeing your photographs, of saying 'I made that'.

These days, I am a middle-aged family man without the time and space to set up a dark room. In the loft I have the equipment - I have promised myself I will make my own prints someday. For now, I pay to have my black and white pictures printed.

What I just wrote may seem technical and dry. It is. I have been criticized by lots of people for not showing, or even having feelings and emotions, but I do have them. I am so passionate about my love of photography and its ability to help me communicate that I am probably repeating myself – another autistic trait. But to be true to you, I must repeat the importance of powerful emotions, allowed a channel to be received after years of denial. To get to these emotions, I frequently need to make a long technical journey and use physical props and do physical things over a long time.

The props and things I do are my way of knowing sentiments, sensations and excitements and, most importantly, giving them a route out. I can talk technically about photography and lots of things - people assume I am being dry. I have been told I have no feelings - that hurts a lot. It's just that when I access feelings and emotions through things and processes, the exact ways these things work is crucial for the process. When going to memories and feelings through photography, the exact way it was done is a key to the really important stuff.

Using a double Gauss or a Tessar, which are different lens designs, makes discernible differences to how images are recorded. This is like the difference in tone produced by different pianos. A trained ear will know the differences between a Steinway and a Broadwood. My wife had a Broadwood, and I have learned the differences. I know how each lens I use will translate the scene in front of me and project it onto the film. My choices are based on my emotional state and how I relate to the subject, time and place. Like musicians feel their emotions through playing music, I feel through making photographs. I'm autistic so I will notice the most subtle details - I'm wired to notice these things. Emotion and feeling will be directed and translated though these things. The finer the emotion, the finer the details will be in our expression. This has nothing to do with being cold and lacking emotion.

I love photographing people; it's the way I can connect with their emotion and make a record of our relationship. I find approaching people hard, so there are not many portraits in my work, but the ones that are there are significant. Most are family, and my relationship with them over the years is in the photographs. One of my favourites is a black and white picture of Joshua, my son. He is laying on the floor, on his front, head up, reading a comic (he was about seven at the time). I lay down at his level and photographed him in his concentration. It depicts the loveliest part of our father and son relationship.

Cameras give me a way of connecting with people, either through the lens in the process of making a portrait photograph, or though conversation. People often ask me about my cameras and what sort of pictures I make - this provides me with good opening gambits in conversation and meeting people. I use camera as stim (stimulating) objects too. I can get different sensations in my hands from handling them, from sensory seeking pain in the back of my knuckles – this is good when I am anxious or my balance is not great. I turn focus and aperture rings for calmness and balance in thoughts and emotions. I use the forms of cameras and their textures for peace and thought as well. Cameras are good for all this as they are designed to be hand held.

I use heavy cameras with large straps over my shoulders to give deep pressure and proprioceptive feedback, good for balance, body awareness and calmness in public spaces.

Cameras often have LED lights in their viewfinders - I use these for visual stimming. The little lights are like small sweets that go with the clearly framed scenes I am seeing. Life comes together well in a viewfinder; at the moment I am rather liking the viewfinder in a Pentax P30t, but not the orange numbers - the green ones and red mode indicator lights are better. The best viewfinder stim I can get from the P30t is to have the red M for manual lit along with a solid and flashing green shutter speeds lit, I like the 250 and 500 lights best.

Today I carry a camera nearly everywhere; the number of cameras I carry relates to my anxiety on the day. A very anxious day can be a five-camera day, but normally it is two or three cameras. I do not have several cameras hanging round my neck - that would be silly. Instead, they are in my carry bag or in my bicycle bag or the car. I do not normally get them all out, but it's good to know they are there. They are chosen for their stim and calming qualities to match how I am on the day. Each one has its own stim and sensory profile and each one will suit different ways I have of seeing the world during the day.

The sensory properties of cameras vary to hold, to hear and to see. I have over eighty cameras; each one has its use. Most work, though there is a small group of cameras waiting for repair. They are machines and they need maintenance like any other machine. I talk about this on my blog at www.autismlivetraining.com - please take a look.

When my grandmother died the only thing of hers I wanted was her camera, the Super Isolette (the one that hurt her fingers). This is the one I remember her by from that time in the park and occasions since. The Super Isolette is currently awaiting a thorough service. Its oil has dried and it is very stiff to operate, so it will need specialist attention. It has some finely made and unique parts in it; it is easily damaged by someone who does not know how to work on it.

The picture from 1970 is on my desk. I remember that scene like it happened this morning. My face is obscured by the camera, so no change then in the last 43 years. If you want to see the photograph it is on Flickr at http://bit.ly/15l2gBv (Richard Maguire cycle.nut66).

Quiet In The Snow

Lots of snow today; I had the pleasure of walking the dog. It really is a pleasure, out in a winter landscape, wrapped up warm with a lively little terrier for company. First walk out of the day and it is snowing all around me. The snowflakes look like moving fogs when I stop to look at them - falling softly, slowly and driven to movement by light wind.

Colours are muted in this white world. House doors, cars and narrow boats - subdued. The most vibrant reds, blues and greens become saturated in white as light remains perfectly even for a measured time, with the ground becoming nearly as light as the low clouds. Vertical surfaces covered in snow, light from all directions, and a world without shadows.

My coat becomes white in the driving snow. Only Jake, our dog, keeps his colour. He will not let snow settle on his bristly ginger and black coat. Walking out of town along the canal towpath, past the bare poplar trees I perceive silence. All sound is absorbed in the laying and falling snow. The silence is beautiful and tastes so sweet - I want to stay out in this to savour the pure quiet moments. All echoes of our Aylesbury town are hushed to a gentle nothing and even the light wind makes no noise in the snow-damped trees. The snowflakes make a lovely soothing pattering 'ssssssss' kind of noise as they settle around me. My breath makes almost no resonance - the loudest sound around me is the patter of Jake's four feet.

I was in sensory heaven throughout that walk with my dog. My normally overloaded senses were at ease and I drank in the peace - there was no sensory overload or fear reaction at all. My normal sensory world had been suspended. I felt elated in a sublime ecosphere of white. And the bonus is that dogs don't chatter. Odd sounds coming from Jake were his sniffing in the snow – and that gave me peace.

We also wandered into the town centre, along the canal, which was very quiet too. I took lots of photographs of this frozen paradise, streaked with snowflakes in clear crisp air. Frosty narrow boats on icy water - a glimpse of paint reveals an elaborate wooden side panel and the odd black mooring rope brings the boats to life. Swans and ducks crowd around the last patch of clear water with only their splashes indicating that free flowing water lurks beneath. The ducks sound their normal warning signals on Jake's approach, although they are getting used to him and becoming less bothered. Nature's noisy alarm call is today quite comforting to my normally overloaded hearing.

Passing car and buses moved toy-like in the dirty slush, their engines at barely more than tick over - no sharp acceleration or loud exhaust notes... lovely. I did not feel fear at these vehicle noises, nor was my head full of sounds grating, screeching and vibrating as it normally is. My head was clear at peace, mmmm, bliss. This happens very rarely. Normally, I have to fill my head with my own internal thoughts to drown out the thousands of sounds. Best of all, I was not in sensory overload positioning and so started to enjoy my own company. I do not know how to say how lovely this was. I savoured the bliss and wondered if this is what most people feel who are not as sensitive to sound as I am – normal people.

My vision was also not being shocked by overload from scotopic sensitivity. The landscape bereft of angular details - all shades low-key and lovely - meant I could look anywhere without pain and visual confusion. I could take the whole scene in. Oh the freedom to see comfortably!

I stayed out as long as I could, but my dogs' short legs got tired and he was slowing down. We went back home. Going in the house disturbed my senses - back to contrasting colours with added Christmas decorations. The tree, red and silver tinsel, sixty lights, sparkly present wrapping screamed out at me in my line of view. Decorations on the piano and mantelpiece gave little place for my vision to rest. I could see everything in overpowering Technicolor, like an unwelcome dream.

Quiet In The Snow

A few hours later I went out again with Jake, back into the muted world of snow, but it was no longer snowing and the air was clear of snowflakes. Things had more definition as the layers compacted into ice, but everything was still comfortable even though there was a little more noise around since the snow had stopped falling to absorb sound. We stayed out for an hour, drinking in the sensory comfort. When we arrived home again, Jake stayed in his basket - tired out. He looked content too.

I love my wife and adore her company - she is simply wonderful and I regard her as my best friend. Julie noticed I was calm and content after the day out. She wanted to watch a film and asked me to join her cuddled up on the sofa. What a wonderful end to a relaxing and gentle day – the good things in life really do cost nothing. We watched Father of the Bride II, a romantic comedy film and she loved it. I, however, would much rather watch something geographic, factual or scientific. I thought the film was exceptionally boring and predictable, but stuck around to give Julie the companionship she needed and me the time to appreciate how much I respect her. She is gorgeous and I am very blessed to be with her.

At times I found the fast-changing bright scenes of the film start to overload me and almost managed it to the end before having to divert my eyes downwards into our blue carpet to absorb the visionary attack. The Christmas decorations, loud film, bright presents under the tree and noise from TV meant I took my leave fifteen minutes before the end. Julie knew I wouldn't last the whole film and I disappeared to the computer room to be surrounded by low-key stimulation objects of familiarity such as my computer and cameras.

School

Hmm, strange place school. It meant different things with different rules, none of which I really got the hang of. School was a place of mystery and getting told off.

First was Mrs Penny's nursery school. This was in a Catholic Church Hall in the high street and I do not remember ever understanding this school. Mum said something about it doing me good and getting me ready for big school, playing with other children. I had no idea what this would be.

Going there seemed fine, going up the hill and past the food shop, where Mum bought me Jaffa Cakes. With my baby sister in the pram - we went past the fir trees with their funny leaves but I wanted to stop by them, as I liked the texture of the leaves and their shapes. Out into the town we went and over the road to the shops. All quite normal so far - I had gone into town with Mum all my life. Then a strange thing happened, it was all a mystery to me. We turned left, through a gate and across a paved area and into a grey building. Inside was noise like I never heard before, lots of people, hard to discern. The room was tall with high windows. I did recognise the play equipment, the climbing frame, slide, sand box and trikes. I knew trikes - I had one, and they go fast; I wanted to go on one. People told me no, I had no idea why.

That morning lots of things happened that disturbed me. Life until then was quiet, me, Mum, Dad, Nancy and few family friends. My grandparents lived down the hill. The barber gave me sweets, the man in the food shop who smiled at me - life was sorted. People found me odd and cute, which stopped them being too angry.

In Mrs Penny's nursery school none of these niceties happened. Too many children, too much noise, blurs of motion out of which children appeared even when they were still. I remember going every day, feeling bemused and anxious about when I would be told off next. I did not know what was expected of me and how I should behave. The women who ran the nursery school would appear out of the blur and noise with their faces looking strange and they would get hold of me and say, 'No!', Don't be naughty!'

I wandered from table to table, scared, bemused, and hoping I could find something to do that I could get lost in until Mum came to pick me up. Two things were all right - one was the woodwork table. It had a box of wood pieces. We could take some out and make things with the hammers and nails provided. I wanted to make a double decker bus like the ones I rode on with grandma. I always started by making the sides of the upper deck. I did not get further than this as there was never enough time. However, I did like the lady who ran this table. She was kind and calm, she did not tell me off. She said I was clever and that I needed to learn more about woodwork to build my bus. She showed me things, which helped and I liked her.

She gave me time and treated me with warmth. She seemed to believe I was good. Every autistic child needs to know someone like her. In amongst all the confusion, anguish and telling off we need a woodwork lady who is calm and of gentle countenance that can slow things down - who will talk and make sense and not keep changing the subject and rules. Someone who will think and come alongside us, see something of our world say it is good and step in with kind words and actions of encouragement.

I recall the woodwork lady most days of my life and especially when I am doing something practical. Her face, presence and voice reappear like a kind friend; she is still with me. I do not remember faces as a rule, but hers, and her brown hair, is imprinted on my mind. She moved slowly and I could see her in detail.

I did get to go on the trikes. They were fun, they were fast and I could ride around the hall on my own. I remember the rush of the air when I went really fast. That was comfortable - not being bothered by the other children and what might happen if I got involved with them, so often I would be criticised and pushed off activities. I got thrown off the trikes though. I went too fast and was dangerous, they said. I knew I would not hit anyone, I had my routes well planned and I could steer into space. I wanted to avoid people all the time while on the trikes and I loved the movement and sense of peace out there on my own. I did come off a few times when taking corners too fast. I didn't mind; I was investigating the properties of three wheeled vehicles. I did not want to do this in our road as the concrete would hurt, but a wooden floor was different. I just slid when I came off.

I was also investigating the Doppler Effect. When I was out with Mum and my sister I noticed the sound of cars rose when coming towards us and then lowered when going away. I wanted to explore this phenomenon with adults who might help to me understand the effect. They did not and they told me off. When I tried to explain they had no idea what I was on about. They said I was being silly. I knew I had to go fast enough on the trike, make a car noise and people should notice the effect. They did not. I now know that people would not have noticed what I was doing nor the simple way I was investigating the phenomenon I had noticed. A preschool child is not expected to investigate physical phenomena instead of playing with the other children. I have suffered lots of disapproval, when I have been innocently investigating similar things. This hurts, especially when people make fun of me, but I need to do these things as they are part of how I make sense of the world.

I also wanted to move on the trike, movement is so soothing. Many autistic people like to move about their environment frequently and at a good pace, I call it ranging. The trike riding offered such wonderful relief.

Nursery school confused me, and there were some good times with the woodwork lady, but with regard to social and education skills, I learned none. Except perhaps the fact that when away from my family I needed to be quiet and not move. They wanted me to move in ways and with people I did not understand, nor could I wholly comprehend them. The telling off hurt, as I had no idea why I was getting told off. The experience just hurt and drove me deeper into overload and caused me to be frightened of nursery school, but I always went as I was taken there.

I had no idea what to do when school proper started. 'Ouch oh ooh err, what happened?' Mum bought me a jumper and shorts and tried them for fit, whilst complaining about the cost of school uniform. What's that? I had no idea what she was on about. What is a uniform? School means Mrs Penny's at the church hall. Mum sewed up a grey bag for a PE kit - hmmmm? I got plimsolls and shorts to put in it along with a new coat.

Then one day, I was told to get dressed in the uniform (but why?). Mum was concerned as it was my first day at school, not Mrs Penny's, and we walked down a road where someone my Mum knew lived, but we didn't go to their house. Instead, we went through a path in a wood to a place built like lots of bungalows, made of red brick. The big building was called a hall. I was led to a classroom. Lots of children were there. We had a teacher, what's that? I remember the tables. I was told to sit in a chair at a table near the teacher's desk. There were lovely big windows. I saw trees, moving and vivid flat green land outside. Were there any birds in the trees? I like watching birds.

Being seated was great, I could be still and observe. Then disturbing things happened. The other children were even noisier. They poked me, made noises and laughed at me. I realised lots of them had already been in this class so they knew what to do. They found my stillness funny. They wound me up, teased me, and gave me wrong information. Being autistic, I always said what I thought without a hint of irony or a lie - or said nothing fearing people's reaction when they found my straight forward explanation disturbing or puerile.

I thought everyone else was like me and I hated all this interaction with intervention - especially as most of the time the children were blurs of colour and noise. They only coalesced into people when they were still. It was normal for them to pull my hair, shout at me, or insult me. I just could not get a handle on school or anything I was supposed to do. The clothes I wore also confused me. I did not like them. The shirt collar scratched my neck, the wool jumper scratched - I shiver thinking about it now if I remember the times for too long.

The teachers would appear out of the blur suddenly and say things to me, or tell me to go places and do things. I was confused and frightened by the staring adults. Our class teacher was nice, though. She had a fresh attitude to life. She encouraged us to explore our subjects. She got us to grow plants on the windowsill to be used in lessons. We also brewed wine. I can't imagine this going on today in the modern school system, but I liked this connectivity and multi-sensory approach to learning. This bit was really fun. I just got on with learning, the other children were noisy. They did not like the way I got on with learning and said cruel things to me. I preferred to be in my world exploring knowledge, ideas and building concepts. I hated it when a noisy face came in on my peace to say things that I found hard to process and then made fun of me.

However, there was one upside to being interested in learning new things. Other children stopped being cruel at times and wanted to know what I had found out. I learned that, by being clever, I could have some nice contact with other children. Then they bullied me later. Why did they not thank me, or be good to me? I had not learned about inconsistency, using someone, manipulation and hypocrisy. I could not understand these changes of mind and they hurt, causing me to cry a lot. I hated school. I really was not getting the hang of what was going on, or what I needed to do. There was no woodwork lady at this school.

Lunches confused me. We all had to go to the canteen for a 'sitting'. Upper and lower school alternated and this changed from day to day. I could not get the hang of this system at all. I do not remember faces very well, so I had no idea in all that movement and blur who was who, much less who was in the senior school. They laughed and teased me during break times. I had no idea what to do about cruelty. I did not know where cruelty came from in the human psyche. I hated break time where the comfort and order of the class gave way to a frightening swirl of noise, pain and humiliation.

To further complicate this pain and confusion, the playing field was used alternately, senior school one day, primary school the other day, and I could never remember which day was which, so I would gingerly make my way to the field, hoping for some sign that of what day it would be. Maybe a comment from a pupil, an instruction from a teacher, anything to make this clear before I got pilloried and bullied for getting it wrong again. I often stood and cried in a corner, or near a big hedge until the bell went.

A lack of organisational skills and an impaired short-term memory frequently go with autism. Parents and teachers, please don't underestimate how hard school is for autistic children. They may be being quiet - this is often freezing because of fright, sensory overload, anxiety and fear. Quietness may be a sign of hiding fear and all sorts of pain. The autistic child probably does not have the referencing and social skills to speak about what really is the trouble. They will contain this until they blow, maybe years down the line. Quiet does not mean things are OK. We are often playing dead, as a result of adrenalin and overload. We are on our own because we do not understand what is going on and it is just too much to interact with.

We are not being antisocial, we are usually going through a living death until we are back at home and that was my experience. School is normally overload, pain and confusion for autistic children. There are lots of misunderstandings, missed opportunities and comparatively little learning due to all the confusion anger and pain. School is a fog of incomprehension, sudden shocks, disapproval, too many messages, too many people behaving unpredictably, too much noise all contained in a mental fog of overload fear and pain. So much of what happens in school would seem unremarkable to a neuro typical person. They have difficulty seeing what we see. All may be normal and comprehensible. To us it is fearful, incomprehensible, painful and horrid.

Bullies would also wait for me on the path through the woods. They knew it was my only way home and the fact that I walked on my own made me an easy victim. I would be called nasty things - my PE bag pulled from me and thrown around, usually ending up in a muddy puddle. I would be hit and kicked. I had no idea what was going on and how to do anything. I could not even reference this pain to be able to give my parents a coherent account of what happened. I do not think anyone knew how serous this was. I had no framework for making sense of what was happening. All I really knew was that it hurt and I cried. I had no friends.

I remember when these attacks in the woods stopped. My Nan came to pick me up from school. She saw the boys ready to attack me. She shouted at them and made them frightened to go near me. They stopped attacking me in the woods from then on. They just found other places to attack me, nearer the classes. I learned from my Nan that these things could and should be stopped. I thought these things just happened. No one in my family was nasty to me, I just assumed that nasty things happened outside my family and this would be normal and painful.

We moved early the next year and I was sent to a new school. I had some idea what to expect, but this school was just as confusing as the first. It had a big hall and the classrooms were separate and set around the hall, which caused me difficulties as I was not usually sure where my classroom was - they all looked so similar. I became hesitant. I did not remember who my classmates were. I did not know who to follow out of assembly. I often went to the wrong classroom. Children laughed at me, teachers gave me directions and I forgot them. Finding the class was trial and error. This was humiliating and gave the bullies an excuse to have a go at me. I became very frightened of school. School was a place where children attacked me. I kept quiet. I did not know I could or should say anything, or how to say it. I did not have a referencing system or vocabulary for bullying.

Please, parents and teachers - if you have an autistic child in situations like school or clubs, please remember that the novelty and confusion of these places may not be recognised or referenced by the child. If there is not a template for understanding and describing what is going on, the autistic child is very unlikely to be able to understand or give expression to what is going on and ask questions or seek clarification. As I wrote earlier, silence is not normally a good sign. It cannot be assumed that nothing is wrong. You are safer to assume that something *is* wrong and the child cannot reference or express it. Time and quiet are useful for helping an autistic child begin to communicate and reference what is going on. Even if nothing is wrong, the child will appreciate the effort you made to come alongside with love and practical assistance. This will boost confidence and self-worth. It will help with space for comprehension and learning in novel and social situations.

I work like this with adults as well, and they love the time spent. They find this liberating, and are able to find themselves and find their way in life a lot better. They feel great too, and much self-harm, anger and loathing goes away rapidly being replaced with happiness and confidence, with quick and long lasting improvements in behaviour and social skills. I find this approach, along with an unconditional positive regard, is the best of all approaches. It will help knit together and facilitate any other approach used.

Please do not underestimate the trauma of first experiences outside the family. Young autistic children will not be fully comfortable, even with home and family. They will take away understandings and mental frameworks from home to outside situations. The understandings and mental models from home will be non-applicable outside home. Relationships outside are nothing like family. Outside people are faster, more numerous, less predictable, care less, listen less, do more and are more incomprehensible. Out of this incomprehension and mental anguish will come confusing demands, social protocols, rules that cannot be recognised as rules.

The autistic child gets negative vibes and scolded, for what? They will have little or no idea. I remember being sixteen and in sixth form, still unable to comprehend and follow lots of rules, formal or social. School can be a hateful place, full of terror, confusion and pain. The child may be passive at school. I recall how I was - the phrase 'frozen with fear' comes to mind as confusion whirled around me. Most of the time I was passive, submissive, too much so. I did not know what to do, or even that I could do something. However meltdowns did happen. When all this got too much it would take a small thing then I went off with a bang. This became a three monthly cycle, throughout my late primary education and into my mid-twenties. It is painful to recall these years and write about them, as they were horrid. Lots of young people with autism attempt suicide and I am one of them.

School was not universally bad. Some teachers ran their forms and classes with a sense of fun and exploration. In years when I had these teachers, school was okay 'in-class'. The bullies were still present at break times and after school. Two teachers stood out that had a sensitive, avuncular way of running their classes - they had high standards and we worked hard. They could think outside the box. The set up imaginative lessons and there were lots of things to try, do and measure in our classes. Both were great model makers and encouraged us to do the same.

I learned a lot through experimenting with models and pictures and I felt sad that the rest of education was not like this. Many lunchtimes were spent in the classroom making spaceships, cars and pictures. In class, at lunchtime, I felt happy. I had something I was good at to do with my time. Other children saw I was good at practical things and were nice to me. That gave me an immense sense of belonging – something that was alien to me. These were the times when I could share and have relationships with my classmates – I can count them on both hands. Normal children can relive these days with time spent in friendship groups as a regular occurrence throughout childhood.

I loved science at secondary school and joined a lunchtime science club. I was very good at making experiments, finding out how to get answers on what we needed to know by being analytically quizzical on minor but important technicalities. I also liked the art club, and was delighted to discover I have a natural creative ability that would later emerge in photographic hobby. I have an instinctive understanding of colour and form and space. My clumsiness did not matter here, I could use this to create texture, and it felt so liberating.

Art club was somewhere to meet the more eccentric pupils who would talk of interesting things and weigh up issues. I loved art club but was unable to continue friendships outside of this environment since the maintenance of relationships based on group acquaintances were a mystery to me. I did not know how to join the artistic crowd - their ways were different from the culture I had at home, yet I loved the art philosophy - real art for the love of it.

Today, I love meeting artists and listening to them talking about their work. I learn so much about life and being human from them. Their ingenuity is a joy to discover – connecting to someone's passion is one of the best things in my life. At secondary and primary school and in a wider context I was always some way behind my contemporaries at any stage of life, which was painful. Dip into one of the chapters in this book - it explains the details of what is going on in my head if approached by a person to speak with them and you will understand my reluctance to engage with vibrant personalities. Only now, forty years later can I put the mechanisms into place that help me to handle groups of people long enough to ascertain their meanings – let alone their words.

Primary school went by and I attained a tolerable level of functioning. I got used to the ways of school. I learned to make jokes out of my social faux pas and plain idiosyncrasies when 'getting it wrong'. The jokes did not usually work but I was learning.

School

Bullies were an ever-present difficulty. They spotted my naivety
and inept social skills, then set up situations to hurt, embarrass or
frighten me. One boy in junior school got a whole gang together –
he and his bullying tactics were petrifying. He learned that
teachers looked out for me and knew my vulnerability, so would
use the walk home to terrify me. During the schoolday he and his
mates would give me the stare to let me know they would 'get
me' on my way home. It resulted in my not concentrating in class
or eating much lunch, and making a great effort to try to stay in
the building at break times, visibly distressed with the fear.

One day, a guitarist came into the school to give us an afternoon
of guitar music and tell us all about classical guitar playing. Many
of the boys were not interested, but the headmaster said that
there was plenty of sport, which they liked, and musical children
had very little. I thought this was a good idea and said so in class.
The bully and his mates took this as another reason to attack me. I
really wanted to enjoy the beautiful guitar music. I loved learning
about Spanish guitars and someone called Segovia, but a dark
menace flooded my afternoon in the hall and I listened through
muted panic. As long as the guitar man was there I was safe, but
the bullies said I would be beaten up on the way home. No Idle
threat, they had done it before – this time it was worse. They
nursed an increasing anger at being made to do something so
unpleasant like listen to a guitar, and recruited some more boys at
the recital through nudges, whispers and pointing.

I was singled out as the victim and remember putting things away
in my desk, getting my coat and being dismissed from school.
From that moment every step took me closer to danger. The
other boys sped past me. I walked the path round the back of the
infants' school to the gate out into the park, unaware I could go
another way home as this route was my routine and could not be
changed without learning another route. They were in a semi-
circle on the grass either side of the path. I had no way to avoid
them, about fifteen bullies altogether - ready for sport. In my
stricken state I had no idea what to do - I couldn't fight or run. I

had no strategies for dealing with this and I could not imagine why people wanted to be horrible to me.

I walked past them blubbering and crying. Tears in my eyes blurred my vision. Taunts that I did not comprehend came at me from lots of mouths. The gang closed in and I kept walking. Nothing in my life had prepared me for this. They said they would put me in the stream or the pond. This had been tried before, but I had a way of staying on my feet. However, if all these boys tried I would not be strong enough to resist.

Punches landed, dull thuds into my little body and frightened head. Thankfully, some of the blows were attenuated by my parka coat. I kept walking forwards with tears running down the front of my face, snot streaming from my nose. The taunts and physical knocks blurred into one horrible experience. Just like lots of people around me blur when I am experiencing a sensory overload, they blurred to become one big pile of arms legs with heads and clothes but not individual people. I cannot comprehend to any great extent what groups of people do around me – that's true even today, but I can at least understand that it stems from my autistic nature. As a child, I had no idea I was autistic or what it meant. I was simply being picked on for happening to be different. They were the majority and all of them united in hate.

I kept on a forthright course aiming for home since there was nothing else to do. The only response I managed now and then was a feeble 'stop it'. This was treated with derision each time I spoke. I was scared stiff and couldn't muster any other words or any actions. I gave the pond a wide berth, but they did try to push me in the stream. I have long legs and a wide stride that helped me get across the narrow slow flowing stream, but it didn't stop the gang and they scurried over to the other side, trying to regroup for a second go. This pattern of humiliating physical and mental agony lasted until I was about half way home, when the group began to disperse. I opened the back door covered in mud, tears and trauma.

School

I love music, especially the guitar. Very often this painful memory comes back to me when I am enjoying or thinking about guitar music and I visibly shiver. Today, I was listening to Comfortably Numb by Pink Floyd in my car on the way home from work. This memory came back when the guitar solo began, and it still hurts. It was a nasty occasion and not the only one - the walk to and from school became a gauntlet of dread for a long time. It put me off learning and lots of life at home. Events like these were, of course, meltdown fuel.

There is one more thing I want to say about this and other incidents - an autistic child will have difficulty accurately referencing the feelings involved to give a coherent account of such events to parents, teachers and carers. These things are carried deep within the person for many years. The hurt sits heavily inside as shame or pain. I could not explain what happened fully enough to my parents, nor could I raise this at school. The result was that no one took it seriously. I doubt they would have done even if they had known – because of my inability to communicate. I was expected to carry on with a hazardous journey to and from school.

Instead, other explanations were sought for the deterioration in my schoolwork and relationships. I knew these explanations were ridiculously wrong - the main one being that I was lazy, rude and did not try hard enough. I did not have the presence of mind, social skills and eloquence to say what was really happening in ways that the adults in my life would understand and take sufficient notice of.

Please - when autistic children are spluttering or whispering something has happened, or going even more quiet than normal, do take notice and take us seriously. Just because we are not terribly eloquent does not mean a lack of severity is behind what we are saying. We are not neuro typical people and we do not naturally put on a front or get overtly emotional. The lack of obvious emotion at the time is a real problem; people do not compute this and will believe we are not very troubled.

221

The truth is, we are often frozen with terror and cannot manage the outer sign of distress – instead, the emotional bit will explode out of us when we have a meltdown. Get alongside us in these situations. We need a friend, someone to believe us. We cannot get too emotional, cuddly, or cry often, if at all. But we are soft, human vulnerable and hurting in these situations. We need someone to be articulate for us. Someone who will not jump to conclusions, but will help us interpret and express what is going on. Someone who will not make negative judgments if we get tongue-tied and relive events out of order. We have difficulty referencing and when we are hurting it is weaker still. We get in a muddle - so please give us the space and love to help us set things straight. We will feel much better and the emotions and pains that lead to meltdowns will be soothed away. We can grow some confidence and put away fear.

Secondary school loomed in 1978 and I grew evermore fearful, knowing I would have to learn new systems, as it would be very different from primary school. I was also getting nearer to teen age, with changes happening that confused me, and I felt ill equipped for this new body. With childhood running out and a process of growing into adulthood about to start, I felt depressed by this prospect and feared the bigger boys and what hurt they could do to me. I did not know then that I would not be bullied at secondary school. I recall being in Harrogate, in our car going to see my godmother. We drove past the Stray. There were teenage lads goading, bragging and play fighting on the grass. This scene frightened me - I could not then, and still cannot, tell the difference between play fighting and real fighting. Would lads like these beat me up in September?

My Dad saw my fear and told me something of teenage life. He told me about bragging and getting physical as a way of bonding and learning about strength and hierarchies. I understood very little of this and I feared even more that I would be more out of my depth socially at secondary school than I was already. I also felt fear at the possibility of being physical, like these lads were. I

222

don't like unexpected physical contact, it hurts and unnerves me. I spent weeks running over what I saw and trying to get it to make sense, but I was worried.

All the bullying I had been through caused me to hate horror films and suspense. They are too close to my experiences from back then. I like reality in fiction and life to be consistent, so there are no hiding places for my fears. In fact, my years at secondary school were quite peaceful compared to junior school. One lad did try to bully me, and I inadvertently used my physical size - hitting him square on the nose in the PE changing room. What a stroke of luck! I don't know who was more surprised... it certainly shut him up and other lads who I could see mentally lining me up for bullying left me alone.

I liked being able to learn subjects in a specialist way at secondary school. I started out really keen and in the top sets for everything. The level at which they were being taught, and by specialist teachers who liked their subjects, thrilled me. However, this fell apart in the first term. My undiagnosed dyslexia and autism meant that I did not have the organisational and study skills to cope at the top level. I did have the intellect, so this was painful as I knew and loved the subjects, but hardly wrote anything down. A slide into educational ignominy started.

So, I knew I was bright and could naturally take in more of the subjects than my peers. But the frustration and pain felt at not being able to translate this into text, homework and tests led to disappointment from teachers and my parents, and to awkward questions from other pupils, teasing and being left behind. My self-esteem slid, term-by-term, year on year. I hated the thought but my dream of university, the study of a subject I enjoy, expertise and the kudos from being valued at being good at something started slipping. I grasped at straws - imagining I could do the academic work.

The parallel world where I was good at things was my refuge in those dark years. I could drop into it anywhere and at any time. I knew it was fantasy and would never work out in reality. Despite that, the fantasy was much better than reality. I worked hard on ways that I could arrange my deep and far ranging thoughts in a way that would get recognition. I grasped at ways of finding self-esteem. I fantasised about what I could do, the friends I could make and the career I could have. I needed these dreams, I could be happy in them. I was not specific, but I wanted to be an expert at something and earn a living with a skill that would be in demand.

Being good at something and developing expertise is not an unusual way for an autistic person to earn a living. We aren't blessed with the greatest socials skills and means to persuade people. We are good at being useful and at things that are in demand, for example at being computer and I.T. experts. My hopes of getting an interesting career were fading and I feared the future beyond school. I began wanting death - the depression was way deeper than I realised.

Worry and negative feedback were normal. Any reference to my strengths was fleeting, rare and couched in worrying terms. There was hardly anything to feel good about. I tried to get comfort in quiet times and places, and to seek the company of people who were positive about me.

I recall one time in my second year when I felt good. I enjoyed my subjects and was getting the hang of a few pieces of work. I was managing to get on with a couple of school friends and had a little money to buy chocolate in the school youth club. I remember one day at lunchtime. I was eating chocolate and feeling good. I had had a good talk with two friends and I was having some space to cogitate and collect my thoughts before going back to class. I remember having an unusual level of confidence in classes. I got some praise in geology from the teacher. I liked her - we were both keen on geology. We would talk geology and explore the different rocks, processes and chemistries. I was good in geology tests. I liked the systems in the planet and how it is always on the change. I wanted to be a geologist as I liked the thought of fieldwork and being out in the wild with a few other, like-minded people. I had read about the Canadian Geological Survey, where their jobs and way of life attracted me.

I went home happy and got on with tea and my evening as usual. My father was in the kitchen after tea, doing something when I went in for a drink. As I breezed in, he called to me and looked very serious - I knew this would not be good, but what now? He said he found me annoying at home; I did not join in, or do enough. My good day ended – that second of self-esteem killed stone dead. I felt crushed, lonely and no good. That day was the last day I felt any real hope at school and at home – and I can pinpoint it to a specific time and place.

I felt that if my dad was disappointed in me, then I was useless. I felt his judgement rest upon me and became sure I would not be successful at anything - death seemed a lovely way of stopping the pain and having rest. I slunk off to my room and cried. No one else knew. I did not feel they would care. I might be a nuisance if I bothered anyone. Of both my parents, my Dad was the one I felt able to talk to. That evening, I felt I had no one to confide in. Dad found me infuriating. But I tried hard, I really did. Now I know my lack of effectiveness around the house and lack of social skills was due to a poor executive function and poor social skills. I really did try very hard, but it was not effective in other people's eyes. They thought I was being apathetic. I knew they were wrong but I did not have an explanation to offer, or the social skills to convince anyone.

For years after that day I felt no hope.

I tried to get morsels of happiness and relaxation where I could but I could not carry these times of happiness much outside their bounds and stretch them on into the rest of life.

My heart went out of education at this point. I still loved the subjects and wanted to do well. I still nursed something of an ambition to go on to university. I still hoped I might be able to use my intellect to earn a living. I knew people did not normally guess at my intellectual abilities. I understood that most people put on a front, to show their abilities and usefulness. I did not do this. I had no clue what to do. I knew I projected very little of my innate abilities. I did hope that after a time people might become interested in me, take notice and want to know me.

In 1978, before I started at secondary school my parents took me to see a psychologist in London. They knew I was bright, but under performing at school. They wanted to know how bright I was and to find out what was going on. Coincidentally, 1978 was the year Lorna Wing was working on her description of autism after hearing Hans Asperger and reading his work. The information was out there that could be used to diagnose my autism. It was new to psychology then and the whole industry resisted Lorna Wing's work and descriptions of autism for a good few years before recognising it.

The psychologist found an unusually large range of abilities and disabilities in my cognitive functioning. A later psychologist found this too and was interested in reading the previous report. Both said they found the largest range of functioning they had seen in anyone. They even rechecked the results to see if they had got them right. From 1978, I knew I was very intelligent but, at the same time, flawed in some way. I hoped that knowledge of my intelligence would help me, but had no strategies to put this into positive use.

My parents also took me to meetings of the National Association for Gifted Children (NAGC), where I came across children as bright and inquisitive as me. That was great, but I could not make contact with any of them as they belonged to a different culture - it was the same problem I had had at school and I felt like an outsider. I could understand quicker than most about exactly what we were doing in class, but I could not for the life of me put it into practice. For instance, I went to an evening meeting on computers and computing and felt thrilled to be shown a new Commodore Pet personal computer. The speaker explained how computers worked, which I grasped quickly, and had reams of technical computer related questions in my head, but I could not formulate a sentence from the sensory overload around me, or socially interact with the other students because of being autistic.

I felt so outside the group at the NAGC that I did not want to go to many meetings. I felt sad about this and I saw the same pattern of dropping out due to social difficulties. I had seen it before and knew this would hurt my chances in life, but had no explanation for my behaviour. The way I understood it was that for most of my life I was just like everyone else, but not very good at much, and felt like a complete failure most of the time. I hurt deep inside to the pit of my stomach and grieved for missed opportunities on many occasions.

At school there was so much of interest as well as so much hurt and failure. The educational psychologist I saw in adulthood said that my school life was a series of disasters - the exact pattern he had seen in many dyslexic people.

PE (physical education) was a particular horror at school. I was very fit and into exercising through cycling and running. However, being autistic means I had little or no grasp of team games. I did not understand the rules, or how to co-operate in a team. I could not read others on the playing field or read the game. This was not too bad at primary school. Teachers there are not normally big on PE. They would usually design games that were playable by all the class or we would play rounders (it's quite like baseball). In these situations I could step back and ignore the game for most of the time.

Then came PE at secondary school, where it was hell. The changing room was huge and crowded, with lots of opportunities for an autistic adolescent to get into trouble through not knowing the social rules. Showers were horrid. They were a den for bullies, along with being filthy and freezing cold - not a place for a young lad with lots of sensory issues and little in the way of social skills, who was no good at holding his own socially.

Out on the field we played rugby. The contact, cold and extreme levels of social skill needed were a miserable experience. As I am naturally clumsy, I was always dropping the ball. This earned me the collective ire of the rest of my team. In fact, the stage of social development I was at was not adequate for playing team games - rugby was pure misery as was the scene in the changing room afterwards. To say that I hated PE is an understatement. I would often lose sleep over having PE the next day. I would not be able to concentrate properly in class before PE lessons.

One saving grace was that the punishment for misbehaviour in the changing room before a lesson would be to run the cross-country course. I loved cross-country. I had excellent stamina. I love moving, running and being out in the countryside. Autistic people often like being in motion - we run and pace. I am a pacer and runner. I call this practice ranging. Many of the autistic people I work with range to and fro. I walk and range a lot during my working day.

Cross-country was a joy and I did very well. It felt good to beat the lads who normally beat me. I could also clear my head out in the Buckinghamshire countryside, running on my own in school time. I would be way ahead of most of the others in my own space, enjoying the quiet clear air around the school grounds, through fields and along the canal.

Indoor PE was nearly as bad, at least it was inside, and I hated everything that went on. I would be made fun of for being ridiculously skinny and tall. I suffered name-calling and being sneered at, as I was also no good at any gym activities. I fumbled, tripped, stopped and fell all around the gym. Even the teachers made fun of me, which made the situation much worse. No one was keeping a lid on the situation. I was on my own. I do not know how to describe the feeling. I was also unable to say or do anything about it. I had neither the social or communication skills necessary.

One incident in the gym I remember well was when we were doing a circuit, using each piece of equipment in turn. I could do very little and had become used to being made fun of for not having the strength to climb the ropes. I had poor technique and was terrified of heights. On this day, I tried as hard as I could to make way on the ropes but got nowhere fast. No one made much of it as we were going at a pace round the gym. I thought I was fine on this occasion, but had thought too soon.

One of the PE teachers stopped the class and told us to sit. Then I was told to stand. I stood, with no Idea why. Next the teacher spoke to everyone in derisory tones about me being weak and unable to use the ropes. I wanted the ground to open and swallow me as I could feel the derision from the class. Then to my horror I was told to climb the rope, and everyone was asked to watch me fail in the task. I was so shocked that I had no wits left and obediently tried to climb. I put everything into this and strained my arm muscles trying to grip the rope and lift myself up it. I could hear the hall fill with laughter and unkind comments. I knew this teasing would carry on well after the class had finished, but could not believe what was happening at the hands of a teacher. I was filled with anger and humiliation that fuelled inevitable tears. After a while, I let go of the rope and stood still with my head bowed down, avoiding my view of the class and the teacher, wishing the situation was not real.

That gym incident took away from my pitiful amount of dignity and already dangerously low self-esteem. I cannot write properly about what I felt then and feel now about that time, since I was bullied and humiliated by a teacher. I lost so much confidence. The pain went inside and sat there ready to surface at my next meltdown. I even feel furious now, many years later, writing about this. Another effect was that this dented my ability to believe in people of authority or adults in general for that matter. For some years after I found that in social situations where jokes were being made, I assumed they were at my expense. I would lose my temper or destructively meltdown – destroying my things, damaging myself or surroundings. People had no idea why I reacted so aggressively and it took some years to pick this mess apart and do something about it. I still have this difficulty over three decades later.

I hated PE so much that I began to miss school on PE days. I would stay for lessons before PE and lunch. Then before the dreaded PE, I would go to the bicycle sheds, get my bicycle and ride off into the countryside - not straight home so no one could trace me until well after school had finished. I wanted to disappear and be on my own. Another advantage of going missing was a reduction in teasing as I got some 'credibility' for playing truant, especially as my mother was a teacher at the school.

Sports days were usually a slow, painful experience, with me being not much good at anything except maybe distance running, but I was not usually picked for this. I wanted to run 1500 metres where I could settle into a rhythm and pick off the lads who were showing off by going too fast from the beginning. I do remember one 400m race where I got off to a good start. One lad, with a huge ego, could not bear the thought of being passed by me - a friendless skinny boy - so took a tumble on the first bend. It didn't even look convincing, but he achieved sympathy from some of the girls, and I had the satisfaction of knowing he had faked it and was therefore not as invincible as he thought he was.

The best sports day though was a gift of coincidence. In art, we were doing the human body. Our art teacher asked if some of us would take photographs at sports day of people in action. It took a while for this golden opportunity to sink in, but I volunteered and was allowed to spend the day taking pictures and not competing. Bliss, pure bliss, wandering around all day without a teacher telling me what to do and with a camera. I used my dad's Contarex SLR, a huge German camera, really impressive. I even got popular to some extent as lots of the children wanted me to take their pictures. What a happy day. I still have the photos from that day and smile when I see them.

I also saw, and immediately wanted, a camera called an Olympus XA that another boy was using for the art project. I was so taken by its diminutive size, jewel-like lens and beautifully placed controls. The focusing was done with a little tab under the lens and used a rangefinder. It had a sliding cover and looked like a piece of sculpture. It was years before I managed to buy one of my own (I have five in my collection) and I always remember that sports day as a tiny taste of freedom with the added excitement of first seeing one of those little marvels. I have an XA placed by my computer as I am typing this manuscript – it's in a beautiful little Olympus pouch. I keep taking it out to touch the shutter controls and trigger memories of happier times - wonderful.

I tried to make friends through being in the school production for a couple of years. First, I helped make and paint the set for a production of Oliver. I loved this, but was still unable to make friends with anyone, even though I was invited to the after-play party. I refused as I did not have enough confidence and feared being embarrassed by making social faux pas and being out of my depth. The following year, our drama teacher asked me to be in the play 'Oh What a Lovely War' and told me to play a couple of character parts. I was both thrilled and fearful. Thrilled because I would be able to join in with the in crowd. Fearful because I did not know them and might not be able to get to know them properly, or might end up making a fool of myself, or could annoy people by not being able to reciprocate if they made conversation with me.

Feeling brave, I attended a rehearsal in the school day, which went fairly well. I loved being on the stage under the lights, feeling the acting turn me into someone else – just like I did daily in the school. I am a great mimic but not very good at being me. I felt a thrill at being up in front of the hall and dreamed of being there in front of an audience. The teacher said I was very good. WOW! I can still remember this compliment today, when I stand up in front of people, which I do frequently. I am a preacher and take lots of church services. It is strange, but given a structured event I have no fear of being in front of people. I love it, and this gives me an opportunity to be alive and communicate with groups of people. After hours of learning my lines, I cycled to school for the evening rehearsals full of nervous excitement.

This was a group of people I liked and wanted to get to know. I knew I had zero street credibility and was regarded as an outsider, but in this context I was tolerated as part of the production. I also wanted to be good at it in the hope that someone would find me interesting and want something to do with me. By this stage of my life at age fifteen, I was also regularly depressed, fighting negative thoughts about myself and everyone else. I arrived at the rehearsals and went to the back of the hall waiting for my turn to be called up onto the stage. No one talked to me and I was patiently silent.

Others, standing around in groups of friends, talked quietly waiting to be called up. There was a buzz of friendship in the room that I so wanted to be part of, and to be alienated felt completely miserable and sad. After thirty minutes of waiting alone, I made it up to the stage once to go through one of my parts before returning to my isolation at the edge of the hall, without friends as everyone else did. I felt sadness, grief and despair. I felt utterly useless and frightened. Like the situations I so often found myself in, drowning in loneliness was too much and I quietly left the hall to cycle home.

The journey back was profound. Feeling the rejection of everyone weighing heavily on my back as I peddled slowly past the streetlights. Soft tears flowed without sound until I was far away enough to be heard before I could openly cry.

On getting home, I put my bike away and waited a little for my face to return to normal before going in. My parents asked how things went and I said very little in return, which led them to believe I was being rude to them, so I went upstairs to bed. This felt like climbing back into my loneliness and the normal situation of not being able to communicate my feelings to anyone.

The next day, after school, mum asked me what had happened the night before - the production team told her I had left and was missed. I did not know what to say and remained speechless in front of her. It was incredibly difficult being an autistic teenager 28 years away from a diagnosis. I felt depression and anger surface, but put on a placid facial expression and said nothing in reply. Inside I felt sad. I had been missed - someone did value me and my company! How lovely!

Churning this realisation in my matrix suddenly made me feel warm inside but a colder thought followed... how do I cope with this? How do I communicate my gratitude to them and sorrow for leaving. After a while, I retreated into anger. It wasn't anger at people liking me and appreciating my efforts, but a deep anger steeped in the roots of my depression. A bile born of many years, suppressed repeatedly but gnawing at me like a worm in my soul. A despair that had been coming to the fore in recent years, a nihilistic resentment. I wanted to destroy myself for being horrid and not worthy of the space I occupied. A self-loathing hatred of what I was. I cried when out of sight of my parents.

The drama teacher came to my classroom to ask if I wanted to carry on being in the play and I replied an optimistic 'YES!' I really meant it too, as I so wanted my parents to be proud of me for something. I agreed to go to the next evening's rehearsal but felt sadness and fear at the idea of returning. My self-esteem was rock bottom and self-loathing had a strangle hold on me. Still, I went along, determined to fight the fears inside me - this determination sitting on top of a seething cauldron of brooding and self-revulsion. When I did get there, I stayed at the back on the floor as before and waited for my part to be called out. Two forces waged a war inside me - one was the determination to go ahead and beat my demons, the other was a fully operational, solid depression bent on self-destruction. In depths of sorrow I felt compelled to throw this opportunity away and left the building without a word or anyone noticing my tears (I was a master at not being noticed).

The ride home became an atrocious melee of my painful moaning, mixed with poker hot tears – I felt horrible. I knew I could go back and be given a chance to succeed but the anger and depression had the better of me. It had the better of me for several years after this and I still feel awful at betraying the encouragement of that one teacher. I still regret not acting, since it was an ambition of mine. I felt that I could be good at it and find happiness in exploring human life through characters. I understood that I could grow into the person I wanted to be - the other me was a fun person, but the current me was intent on death.

Along with being a mentor for autistic adults and children, nowadays – years later, I preach in my local church, but this does not involve acting. Standing in a pulpit, addressing a congregation means I have to be me, which is something I feel good about today. I was voice and stage trained when training to be a preacher. I have many of the actors' skills and I love it. But that was then and this is now... one of the main reasons I love my calling – helping other autistic people be able to live a happy fulfilling life.

Something else happened while I was at secondary school, which is worth mentioning. My behaviour and moods were causing deep concern to my parents since we had come to a point of little communication. I had meltdowns, they were exasperated and we were becoming further apart. They would not talk to me without arguing or me to them without arguing, or long periods of silence. I was also so far down into my depression that at one point after a particularly horrid meltdown (back then, meltdowns were not understood as they are today), I felt like I was going completely mad. This was the only explanation I had for what I was doing. I felt utterly hopeless and started to wonder if I would be better off out of home and far away from anyone I knew. I wanted to be put into a mental hospital. I hated the idea but believed I was no good to anyone. I desperately wanted to be sectioned.

My parents were at their wits end and called the doctors surgery. Two doctors came out to see me - one was a new doctor taking over from the doctor I had grown up with for years. This doctor is my GP (General Practitioner) now, and I can honestly say that she recognises how to heal and deal with things in a balanced way. They both agreed that sectioning was not the way forward for me and it gave me some hope (underpinned by fear) for my future as I was sure I could not make it in the 'normal' world.

One outcome of the meeting with both doctors was to refer me to a child guidance centre but it proved as useful as a chocolate teapot. I smile now, recalling sessions in centre - sitting as a family! This approach didn't work since I would never speak properly of what was bothering me. I had yet more appointments with a child psychologist.

The first appointment went well, because he asked lots of questions about my life and what was important to me. I hoped it would go somewhere - maybe he could help me make sense of what was happening and I could get a grip on everything including happiness. On subsequent appointments he said almost nothing – remaining silent for the whole hour. I had no idea why and was incapable of opening a conversation. Sometimes I dug deep and tried but he went silent again. I thought this was odd and a little creepy. I did go for lots of sessions, though, since they were on Thursday afternoon, when I was due in rugby training. What a fantastic 'get out of jail free card' - I used it for nearly a term. The sports teacher asked me if missing PE would injure my fitness and health. My reply was one of the best I have ever given. 'I cycle over five miles from the school to the clinic and then cycle home again after cycling to school in the morning'. He had nothing else to say to that.

I did stop going to the centre after a while though as couldn't stand much more of sitting in brightly lit, starkly furnished room, staring at a creepy bearded man who made no effort to help me. He would look at me and breathe from behind his beard. I stopped going after waves of despondency flooded my head and I began to feel he was letting me down. I had hoped this would work and I would get some clue as to how to get on happily with life. Sadly though, no one knew much about autism. There were also no interventions for someone like me. I don't even think autism was recognised outside a few people leading medical research at the time.

I remember my last session at the clinic passed in complete silence. I was increasingly upset with ever second passing and the cavernous pessimism returned. My life was still going nowhere fast - a couple of months seems like a very long time to a teenager. I felt betrayed and miserable so left early without saying a word to the psychologist. I just stood up and left his unwelcoming room. On the way out, instead of confirming next week's appointment with the receptionist, I said I would not be coming back at all. She didn't even look surprised. I hoped she would speak to me to ask why - a friendly or concerned voice would have meant lots at that moment and may have even convinced me to stay. Unlocking my bike to cycle home was yet another admission of failure. I felt sad because something I had pinned my hopes on did not work out. It would be back to my miserable life as normal, including rugby training on Thursday afternoons.

I wanted some sort of understanding from these sessions and a way forward. Confidence and social skills training would have been great. A friend to confide in...

I carried on through secondary school in a muddled sort of way. I did well in some places, such as technical design, but was desperately behind in others. I was never popular, although I did gain respect from my knowledge of bike maintenance in the bike sheds at break times. The bike-shed group was made up of people who found mainstream life at school hard. Sometimes one of the popular children would come down to the bike sheds when they needed to talk – I simply fixed bikes and became a listening ear for a precious moment before being ignored again in the classroom. Strangely enough, these incongruous times helped me to hang in with living and stay at school until the age of sixteen to take my exams.

I did try to the best of my abilities. I really wanted to succeed. I still nursed a hope that I might get to university. I tried hard hoping for a breakthrough that may lead to academic success. Maybe my talents could be spotted and someone would believe in me. Maybe there would be some way, maybe. This little hope kept me going through dark times and hard criticisms. I knew I was bright, but could not find a way of connecting with formal learning and showing I could get into higher education and an interesting job. I so wanted to be free to use my mind. So far all I could do was plod, mess up and appear uninterested. I also had no way of referencing and expressing my feelings and aspirations. I could talk about technical things, but not feelings. I felt silly for harbouring my aspirations, knowing there would be no realistic way of meeting them when I feared criticism and derision from people around me if I said what was in my heart.

I did take my exams and emerged with a handful of passes. I spent my summer holiday that year mostly out on my bicycle and thinking about sixth form. I achieved those exam results through a passion for the subjects and an obsessive matrix modelled memory. Coursework did not have a great deal to do with it.

Sixth form started with a new uniform, a common room and fewer fellow students. I had been determined to stay on at school to the age of eighteen since junior school. There was a new social life in the sixth form. I mostly stayed in the fringes of safe distance and talked technicalities of design with anyone interested.

Part of sixth form life was carrying out duties around the school and I was very keen to do these. The word 'Prefect' was, and still is, a dirty word for me. I was keen to do things with a sense of justice (key autistic motivator), but every day I became muddled and missed an opportunity to understand an action. There was a rota system displayed on the common room wall that I read and promptly forgot. I also struggled with studying at A-level standard since the rules were different - I had to co-ordinate more, use more sources and apply quiet time disciplines for self-directed study.

I had no preparation for these new ways of study. I could be good at them if I had time to build up cognitive templates and learn a way of co-ordinating what I did or was expected of me, but the quiet time for study was not quiet for me. I am hypersensitive and have difficulty concentrating if there is any sort of stimuli. I cannot turn my attention away from so many things in an immediate environment. Study time was spent worrying, looking out of windows, with my mind wandering and getting hardly anything done. Teachers began being concerned that I was going to classes under prepared. I often looked foolish and lazy. I was aware of concern, of course but I did not have the social and communication skills to sort things out and raise the right issues with the right people including my parents.

I slipped and slid through my first two weeks at sixth form, feeling my confidence disappear, but put a brave face on and kept going while knowing I was going nowhere. I pretended I was tired of school and wanted to try myself out in the world. Other people in the common room began to notice I was often getting into trouble out of anger and frustration and expressed their concerns.

One wet and windy Thursday morning, word got out that the Deputy Head wanted to see me. Others in the common room knew something was up. My dejection such that I was beyond help that morning. Mr Smith said the deputy wanted to see me in his office – outlining discussing me not trying or doing enough. I found co-ordinating learning and these new duties impossible to combine as I have significant impairments of function. No one knew that then though.

I went, sick with worry to the Deputy Head's office. He had a fierce reputation and called me inside with a sharp tongue, making me stand on the carpet some distance from his desk. His recitation of the list of my failings collapsed my hopes of surviving. I listened to his conclusion - I was a bad, lazy student and a disgrace to the school. I wanted the floor to open and swallow me, but instead slumped my shoulders as I retreated deep inside my soul, leaving only a breathing body visible on the outside. Standing there, I silently screamed at him that I did want to do well, but could offer no explanation or defence that he would find credible. I had tried to explain myself to people over the years, but they treated what I said with incomprehension, disbelief or a contention that I was offering excuses. I know now that I was trying to explain autism. Back in 1982 there could only have been a handful of people who could have recognised my description.

The Deputy Head's next question took me by surprise. He asked if I wanted to remain a pupil at the school, was I even interested in education, as it would be a waste of his time to continue bothering with me unless I bucked up my ideas. I wanted this horrid situation to end that second. My mind hurt and raced when faced with questions and criticism. I had no coherent thoughts to hand. Inside I welled up with anger, grief and a sense of self-destruction, I wanted to die. All my hopes crashed and burned in that office. I guessed it was no use saying I would try to do better, as I would still have the same difficulties with organisation and duties. If I said I would do better I suppose I could have lasted another week before appearing in the same office staring at the same patch of carpet. So, I said I did not want to continue at school but I did not mean this for one minute and I hated saying it. Deep down, though, I could see no other course of action in the circumstances. I felt so hopeless - a desperate and lonely feeling. He said that as I was sixteen and could not be made to stay at school any longer... I had better go. That was the end of school.

I walked out, feeling like I was dying, blinking away tears stabbing at my eyes. I collected my bicycle for the last time and set off home, grieving for the lost promise I made to myself in junior school. Tears ran freely down my face as I peddled faster, remembering my mum's happy face when I said I would work hard at school, stay until I was eighteen and get good qualifications. The memory slapped my cheek hard and I closed off the memory to my mum's smiling face. She was still teaching at the school I had walked away from, blissfully unaware of what had happened. I rode home in my uniform for the last time, sobbing with wretched gasps at life.

At home I changed into casual clothes and felt quite wretched until mum walked in, visibly upset. She never said a word. We knew the real storm would come when my dad got home. And it did, at teatime. Dad let mum tell him I had left school, her voice cracked with the strain of being close to tears. Dad went apoplectic with rage at me, and there was no way on this horrid planet I could begin to explain what the problem was when his furious demands for an explanation came spitting into my face. I was far too upset and frightened, and sobbed I had had enough of school. But that was not the truth. I would have returned the next day if it wasn't for the same destructive sequence of events repeating itself, exhausting me mentally and physically in the process. I resigned myself to school having ended that day. I cried when no one could see me.

Dad said I would have to go and get a job the very next day and pay my way as I would not be supported doing nothing. I was scared of what the future held for me – aware I had no chance of a decent job. I also knew I did not have the social skills or self-confidence to succeed in work. I was incredibly depressed, but had no idea of the gravity of my depression. I became angry and just said I was fed up with school - that was the anger speaking. I did know how to take the next step in my life at that time. My inability to define and explain my difficulties compounded my incomprehension and fear. I was left with putting on a front and pretending I could do something. The bottom had fallen out of my world. My ambitions were unobtainable and I saw no hope for the future.

For the first time in my life, I contemplated suicide.

The following morning, my mum said she had come up with a plan. I could try to take my A levels at college. She thought I needed a new environment and different learning culture. Anything sounded good to me and I agreed to go with her for enrolment details (see chapter titled 'College').

Sensory Overload

I have gone into sensory overload today. It's an unpleasant and unwelcome experience. My hearing was the main sense burning at me, although others cut in after a while. I can keep up a pretence and appear to be functioning, but everything inside me operates as if on an emergency drill - running to keep me upright and conscious. I still respond to people but the pain of responding is unbearable. All my senses are on fire, especially my hearing, which gets affected by tinnitus.

The result is a sensory meltdown and an inability to carry on. Riding my bicycle helps to restore the balance between me and the world, as does menial tasks like errand running that doesn't involve interacting with another human. After occupying my mind with mundane tasks, I cleaned the kitchen to perfection and mentally switched off my brain chatter channel. I am recovering a little now. Life with autism can get painful at times. One trouble I have found over the years is that I look 'normal' and most people expect 'normal' behaviour from me all times. As a result, I am rarely able to kick back and be my autistic self.

The Pentax 'ME' Super

Associations and memories are anchored very strongly in autistic people. For me, they are like way markers in my life, as they feed my complex emotional processing – good and bad. In the countless bad times amid confusion, I cling to good memories - feeling the calming sensations wash over me again and again. This is a wonderful feeling as most of the time I cannot feel any emotion except anxiety. In my reflective state, memories are visual and often become bathed in a golden evening-type light. They include new insights into the situation I encountered and I can literally taste the sweet flavour of pleasure in a rare moment of hope.

In my teens I felt horrid, knowing I was an underachiever and not getting along with other people. I had no idea how I would build a future and live as an adult. Most of the time it all felt hopeless and I survived each day at a time, scared of getting older. What kept me going were the sporadic bright moments, a handful of good occasions and the rare successful connections with people in one to one situations. These erratic lovely times were when, just for a while, I found acceptance and an association with the world – standing in my own goodness to join that value with the goodness in others. These were sweet, scarce times with people I had a common interest with, such as bike maintenance or photography. In later life, I now know this is the way many autistic people find friends - through shared interests.

The Pentax ME Super plays a part of one of the good periods when I made friends on a holiday. Before I go on it is important to know what a Pentax ME Super is. In autism, all the details are important, and in this story the ME Super is a specific detail. The Pentax ME Super is an interchangeable lens single lens reflex camera. Things will get technical for a bit, but stay with this and you will learn something of the autistic mind that relates to and collects details.

The ME Super is a development of the Pentax ME. The ME was launched in 1977 as an aperture priority automatic camera. It was also an important development of the move towards miniaturisation that was happening in SLR 35mm camera design in the 1970's. The camera that started this trend was the Olympus OM-1 launched in 1972. Pentax shaved a millimetre or two off the size of the OM Olympus cameras for the M series of Pentax Cameras. The ME Super added manual exposure to the ME design and was launched in 1978. It also pioneered push button control, combined with a mode dial for operation of the camera. Given the siting of the mode dial, there is not room on the top plate for a traditional shutter speed dial. In the viewfinder, a row of LED's indicted the shutter speed set and over or under exposure indication in manual mode.

In reviews of the ME Super from 1978, testers were amazed at the accuracy of the shutter and consistence of operation. It also had a top shutter speed of 1/2000th of a second, a headline feature in its time. Also this 1/2000th speed was accurate and consistent due to being electronically timed. The push buttons were a unique feature and contributed to sales. The ME Super was the talk of camera clubs and columns in photographic magazines. All over the world of photography, people peered at and prodded these buttons and remarked on the future of camera design. Some said they were not as good or as intuitive as a dial, others liked the simplicity and accuracy of the system.

The ME Super also had an innovative easy loading system, involving plastic rollers that gripped the film end on loading, much easier than locating sprocket holes. It also had a film advance indicator on the rear just under the wind on lever. These features are important, since one of the main causes of not getting pictures on a film camera is misloading the film, which causes the film not to advance. The ME Super was simplicity, reliability and accuracy all rolled into one of the smallest 35mm SLRs yet seen. And if you have not used one they are a series of tactile delights to use; smooth, quiet and with a reassuring quality feel.

If you go on the internet and search for Pentax ME Super you will see pictures and read what photographers say about them today.

You will find a lot of articles, videos and blogs all rooted in autism about the Pentax ME Super.

That brings me to some golden memories. It was 1980 and I was fourteen and on my first holiday away from home on my own. I was, and still am, a keen cyclist. On this holiday I was staying at a place called Loosehill Hall, a study centre in the Peak District National Park in England. I went on a week-long cycling holiday to get 'away from it all', and it is a lovely way for an autistic person to holiday - with people who have shared interests. That week was bliss - I met like-minded individuals and cycled with them all week long. I remember the lady who led the week's activities, and also a French couple from Normandy. We talked about bikes for hours.

All the people admired English bicycle design and became very technical in discussions - a great autism-friendly discussion. We rode out on lovely routes previously researched by our leader in a scenic part of England. I can still recall the warm sunshine, the deep textures and colours of passing trees, grass growing in limestone countryside. The incredibly different dark and light shades of moorland, coming into view as we travelled in a pack like procession, cycling across unforgiving mountainous peaks, will stay with me forever. I will also savour the memory of swimming in the River Derwent, just above the rebuilt pack horse bridge at Slippery Stones. I can recall the well dressings there in intricate detail and so enjoyed photographing them. I still have the pictures somewhere from this holiday, they are my priceless treasures signifying hope.

In the evenings we would meet the people who were on a week-long photography holiday. I was in autistic passionate interest heaven. In the evenings, they showed the slides they had taken and talked photography. It was on these evenings that the Pentax ME Super was discussed. I had not heard of it or seen one before. That year I was using my first SLR camera, a Pentax K1000, and was full of photographic possibilities. I bought it in Aylesbury for one hundred pounds and three pence - earning the money by repairing bicycles in a local shop. I still have that camera thirty years later and it remains in pristine condition.

During those lovely evenings on holiday, the ME Super became the reference point on which I fixed my memories. I am autistic, remember, and anything I am interested in will be a huge reference in any part of my life.

The holiday was special to me because I was accepted just as I was, something that remained unusual in my life then. I was far more accustomed to being on the outside of all company and very familiar with feeling as if I were in the wilderness - away from friendly human contact. So, you can imagine the deep feeling of joy I experienced as I talked, joked and shared a passion for photography. These men were all middle aged and I always felt more comfortable with people who were older than me. I liked their longer and wiser view on life. They were not interested in fashion, like my teenage peers (I was fourteen) and I spent hours listening to their wisdom. Later, I learned that autistic young people often like socialising with adults, avoiding the instant judgement of young people. As I had sought out a holiday that suited my obsessions and did it as a teenager, I simply had not idea I was making friends with men three times my age - I craved kindness. Age, fashion and culture make very little difference to me.

Whilst I shared rich discussions, jokes and anecdotes with these adult men, I learned more about photography than I thought possible, I think they liked sharing their passion with an interested young person. Knowing what I do now about autism and obsessive interests lends me to must that there was a lot of autism in that eclectic group of people. Nowadays, I see many signs of autism in the photographic world, usually amongst undiagnosed middle-aged men in technical jobs that utilise the company of other photographers. Their wives are rarely present at group or club level gatherings and they speak humorously of spousal disapproval with regard to the time and money they spent on photography. By the way, this is my situation today and I am delighted to say I'm a very happily married middle-aged photography enthusiast who believed he would be no use to anyone, destined to suffer a terrible depression caused by autism.

I have never forgotten that holiday when for one whole week I was accepted just as I was. I had not experienced that depth of company and friendship before. The memory is one of the things that carries me through the sad times and I have had many miserable years in the last three decades. These memories hang in my head like a talisman - lifting my mood and feelings. I can recall when I was liked for being me – autistic, different, awkward, confused, obsessive, paranoid, loving, angry, and euphoric with an open heart that is so easily crushed by narrow-minded individuals. In my lowest times these memories kept a glimmer of hope alive in me that I could have friends and happiness, albeit with autistic obsessive wonderful bunch of adults at a camera club, or a dedicated cycling holiday.

These memories also focussed my anxiety when growing up worrying that I would not manage in adult life. For that week in 1980, people responded to me as a liked and competent young man. My intelligence was recognised and commented on. Can you imagine my headmaster's response! And here I was, with my peers, in terms of interest and culture. I knew that these adults had interesting careers using technical ability at which they were competent and valued. They made their living being good at something. Oh wow! What fantastic news was that! I, however, was approaching adulthood with a weight of dread in my stomach wondering what I could possibly do – everyone I had met so far had told me I was stupid.

I knew I was intelligent and keen to learn but this had no form or focus that I could detect. My academic work at school was poor and people around me expressed concern over my lack of progress, which confounded my feelings of fear. Nothing had coalesced in the many disconnected thoughts I had that could be regarded as an aspiration with regard to a profession or career. I was just not achieving for reasons I did not know. But that week in

1980 showed me that there was something there, within me that had potential... as yet indefinable.

The Pentax ME Super has stayed in the fulfilling part of my memory matrix. The thought of it sometimes makes me laugh out loud or smile instantly if relieved in the supermarket or walking down the street. Last year, an ME Super was for sale in a local charity shop. I did the nearest thing an autistic person can do to buying on impulse. I went in the shop, asked to see the ME Super and started at it for a while. I handled the casing and spent a few minutes in a reverie of at audible memory events and personal successes.

I stayed in that state for a while then said as if from a deep place in my soul 'I'll have it'. I have not parted with money so happily for a long time and carried it out in a plastic bag eager to get home where I could explore it in greater depth and load a film. It has been in constant use since and is a delight to operate - I take pictures with it today, recalling the slide projections I saw in 1980. It is a little piece of happiness hanging from my neck when I go out, it goes everywhere with me.

Work

I have learned more about life at work than anywhere else. Here is something I wrote for The Autism Hangout site...

I have seen work and autism go so well together. Work is something that goes beyond an autistic's obsessively passionate, and often narrow, interests. Work requires commitment, humility and team working - going outside of what we would normally do. Work rounds us out and teaches us to deal with life and people, using what level of skills we offer. We also have to be responsible for ourselves and motivate ourselves. Work is engaging, but not necessarily fun. It follows someone else's agenda - that of the business and not of our own. We autistic people can be too narrow at times and this is so needed to round us out.

I often see young autistic people who have been through a special education system who are poorly prepared for interacting with unfamiliar people – especially the skills needed to respond socially in situations as a non-autistic person expects. Work puts us in contact with people we might not otherwise meet or get to know. Work requires us to get on with everyone in the world of work around us. We must also work on a shared process, given to us not generated from within. I have not seen anything else so effective in the autistic life for getting us out into the world and getting on with people.

Many autistic people have come on in life through work (me included), as it makes use of a skill. It can help us through our hardest times, such as bouts of depression or suicidal thoughts. I do not think I would be here today if I had not worked when I was younger; the daily activity and commitment of the work environment did a lot to keep me active and alive. Work gives us something to get out for, a means of meeting and interacting with people and something to be good at. Work gives us little victories each day we work - life becomes less hopeless when this happens. Work makes our brains and bodies work. Crucially, for autistic people, work widens our vision and gets us to interact and observe social skills.

It has been said that whatever works for autistic people, also works for learning-disabled people. I believe this to be true and it is integral to my working life. I have known and worked with hundreds of learning-disabled people - they all want to work and do something useful at whatever level they are capable of. Everyone is skilled - all that is needed is help to find their skills and feel confident in using them, as well as an opportunity to work. Opportunities are hard to find if one is learning-disabled and/or autistic. However, I would always advise people to go for opportunities and encourage making them happen.

The best times I have ever had working with learning-disabled people have been connected with work. For ten years I worked with learning disabled people on conservation and wildlife habitat maintenance. Kinaesthetic learning in an outdoor environment works so well; everyone found his or her level of competence naturally. They won a lot of respect from local people, who liked the work they did and the natural areas they were maintaining. This means so much more than praise from someone who is paid to work with them or any rewards system. It was genuine too, and not contrived. No one had to like them, or be thankful for what they did. They were simply there because of the workload and everyone's personal qualities.

I see the same positive situations happening with autistic people without learning disabilities. In my wife's daytime service, www.seestheday.org.uk, learning-disabled people run a coffee shop. They do this well and everyone has something they are good at. They are not just recipients, they offer something to people by working. I cannot say enough how useful and good this is.

People need a chance to develop. Work does this. It has a purpose and needs to be structured properly. A structure is very useful for anyone who is learning disabled and/or autistic. Often a simple, low status job is all that's needed initially. These jobs teach humility and commitment, while helping people learn social interaction, being part of a common purpose with other people. I so often see these skills and attitudes missing in too many autistic people. However, they are normally present in learning-disabled people with or without autism.

I began work pumping petrol on a forecourt - a simple job that allowed me to gather an observational understanding of the social niceties needed in life and work. I moved into a series of low status jobs after that, and disliked most of them, but I learned slowly and did better in every job I had. I picked up so much about life, people and who I am in these menial jobs. I call them the 'long apprenticeship'. In my current role, I action all sorts of motivating management decisions on issues in the world of autism. Today, work is rewarding and I am respected for what I do, but I would never have achieved my current status without all the tiny details learned in low status employment. As an autistic adult, I am glad I spent the time learning humility, kindness and my place in the world through insignificant roles. Other autistic people have done this too.

Work is hard to find for autistic people. We are the most under-employed group of adults in the world. Even if paid employment is not available, volunteering is a good way to help build up skills, self-esteem, a CV of commitment and experience for a paid job. I would also advise autistic people to do something out of line with their passionate autistic interests. Going outside of an obsession widens thought patterns and teaches valuable life skills in the process. There is more to life than our special interests and we need to know this in order to be of reliable value. Work is not about fun or leisure and that is a lesson too. We can learn about mannerisms, productivity, thresholds and many other things if we start to become a part of society in low taxing roles.

The above is based on my life and the work I have done with young autistic adults over the last 25 years. Life beyond education is something we need a lot of preparation for. I am going to a school next week to spend time with a group of teenage pupils on preparation for life after education. A farsighted teacher knows this preparation is desperately needed, and I am concerned that too much autism specific education gives autistic students absolutely no idea of what they will face when they leave school. I have worked with many autistic adults who were ridiculously unprepared for life and work beyond school and became terrified of making the step into normal society.

In theory, employers should be sensitive and supportive of diversity. In a lot of countries this is legislated for too, but in real life it's very rare. The working world is set up for neuro typical people. That poses autistic people a huge set of challenges in a) getting and b) keeping jobs. I see a lot of young people emerging from education with no understanding of this at all. Either they have unreal expectations that they will be treated the same as they were at school (especially if they went to an autism specific school), or they have been frightened and feel overwhelmed. They know the support they have been accustomed to will cease on finishing school. How will they cope and what will they do?

I remember being nineteen and leaving the education system. It was one of the darkest times in my life. I had no idea how I would get on in society and felt a sense of loss and grief at having no perceptible future. Knowing my peers had advanced much further in life was a crushing blow - I was way behind them. Life felt hopeless and not worth living. I was bright and had plenty to offer, but just could not put that to positive use. Instead I felt convinced that because of my 'oddity' I had no real value and I did not deserve to exist. There was no one to talk to about this, as autism had not been 'discovered', I just bottled it up and carried on in a horrid hopeless life. I use this experience a lot in my work mentoring autistic adults and I help the people around them to understand their situation. Most importantly, I help these individuals – employers, friends, family, colleagues who encounter autistic people in their work respond with kindness and understanding.

Imagine having lots of potential and not even being able to connect with it. Like being a Coke bottle all shaken up - full of pressure with the lid still on. Imagine not even knowing the lid is on or that it could be removed to let the energy inside out. Imagine the nihilistic loneliness gnawing away at oneself resulting in a desire to self-destruct. I do not know any way expressive enough with words to communicate how bad this feeling is in an autistic person's life. This feeling drives a lot of depression and suicide in young autistic lives. They have nowhere to go, no reason to live and no hope. Death seems like the only place to get some peace and it becomes an attractive option. The only form of control left, the only plan available. I was in that place.

Working in mundane jobs, alongside my interests (one of which was cycling) got me through life day by day. If you don't have any hope, you keep going through the motions, unaware events could get better. I had no idea how to proceed, or any hope that these low paid jobs would work in my favour, but they gave me a reason to get up and do something. They gave me a structure and way of meeting people, a way to feel like a human, with something positive to do.

My early jobs were simple ones that just required me to have physical strength and to follow instructions. That was enough, although I felt a strong sense of grief at what might have been, if I could have accessed education. I recall working in a DIY store. I hated that job because of the manager and his attitude. He was a bully. I spotted him straight away. I knew a lot about bullies. I remember imagining where I would be, if I were on a degree course. I dreamed about the interesting people I would meet, the things I would learn and what it would be like to live in expectation of an interesting career. I wanted to use my mind. I tried, but had no outlet. Would life be like this all along? I feared it would.

I had grown up in a middle class culture that put academic achievement at the top of all human endeavours. This achievement, I had been told, would help me have a happy and prosperous life and enable me to live in a big house. The house was not important, but the fulfilment was.

I often come into autistic people's lives at this point, this very point in their lives, through my current line of work as an autistic mentor. What I do is listen to them, reassure them they are not alone and that they are clever, loved and talented. I show them exactly how they have a purpose in life, and that at their young age it is normal to still be exploring and not yet know what direction they would take. Some autistic people already have an aspiration to follow a life path, a direction, which is good, but they need help with making plans to get this implemented.

They also need to be realistic - they will not hit the top straight away. Many think, just because they are intelligent and driven, that should have a place of respectability in their choice of career tomorrow. I explain how careers are built and how proving one's self, learning from mistakes and making connections lead to getting to a good footing in a chosen field. I help them understand that getting on with people and building up networks is more fulfilling than shooting for the top with no network of colleagues or friends to fall back on. They often do not know this, and have no plan of how they will achieve their ambitions. I also help people see that they can make profound changes to their ambitions if they decide something they wanted to do is no longer right for them. Many people feel constrained to stay limited within the strict bounds they thought were good for them - often decades ago in their early lives.

For the people with no hope, of which I was one, I help them know it is possible to develop careers and new directions in their lives at any time. An essential element for developing hope in the autistic life is to have a plan and understand how it can be structured. It helps to show people how to replan their lives, in order to lead to a better future. This works with learning-disabled people too. They want to be successful in their lives, but have often have been told quite firmly by people at many points along the journey of growing up that they will achieve nothing, both overtly and by implication.

Work

The saying 'give a man a fish and he will eat for a day; teach him to fish and he will eat for life' works well as an analogy for teaching and mentoring autistic people. One can say 'plan for an autistic person today and they will cope with today. Teach them to plan and they can plan for life'. Planning is important for us autistics - we are bottom up detail thinkers, to paraphrase Temple Grandin. That sort of thinking is a good discipline and thorough, however we are not often able to see the bigger picture unless someone tells us how. When we have this skill, our lives can progress as we have a valuable concept in which to fit our detailed thoughts and insights. Only when we grasp this can we plan and develop hope for the future. This can be taught at any time but the earlier the better; work hones this skill and adds more skills too.

I worked in a cycle shop, repairing bicycles, which should have been perfect, but it only lasted for eight weeks. I was good at fixing bikes, but at fifteen I had not developed enough social skills to get along in a daily work environment. One thing I remember being in charge of involved fixing punctures - the shop owner said she thought it would be better to replace an inner tube than to repair one. Up until then, the practice was to make a repair. I thought she was voicing her thoughts and did not realise she was giving an instruction.

It was implied meaning that caught me out - being autistic, I do not comprehend implied meanings, I hear words and process them literally. Later in life, I grew aware of looking out for these indirect communication traits to try and guess someone's alternative meaning. I frequently do not get it right and lots of the time, I really am guessing (ask my incredibly patient wife). If my boss at the bicycle shop had said 'change inner tubes from now on' I would have done just that. So I was told to leave because she thought I did not follow orders.

Working

Unemployed and relying on benefits in 1988 was morale destroying. I had been working as a student nurse in Wales. That had been my big effort at striking out and making a life for myself. It was my first attempt at living away from home and I was following my passion for helping learning-disabled people. I had also worked for a while as a nursing assistant in a hospital near to my parents' house. I loved the people - they showed me so much about life and relationships.

A learning-disabled person has a reduced capacity to intellectualise life and consequently a greater ability to live a life of a trust in a simple and happy nature. Learning-disabled people taught me how to relate to a people - with them, I saw how to discern a person's soul. It was good to know that what I suspected naturally actually did lie at the heart of a person - the genuine self, unaffected by clutter or damage. I can see a character's intentions and understand if they are pure. That is the level on which I want to relate to all people because it feels natural, simple, sweet, powerful and humbling.

Learning-disabled people take a while to trust you, and as they are searching your psyche to find out what your intention is, they innocently look right into your soul. It's quite disarming if you are not used to it. Many of the learning-disabled individuals I have met over the years have done this extraordinary practise without words, and they will communicate to you your innermost life. Your own soul and intentions had better be true, because if it is not, that knowledge will be communicated back to you, and all of this is done without words.

I have mentored many student nurses in my career, and on their arrival at work I tell them about this incredible ability clients have to ascertain intentions. I forewarn them about the searching power of a learning disabled person's perception and truthful communication. I say they will connect with you in 'pure human' whether they are verbal or not.

Responses vary from knowing it all 'been there and seen that' to completely sceptical with added humour. At the end of the first week in the placement of care, the students know what I am talking about - they have been regarded purely as humans and not for any affectation or ability. The quality of their personality shows in these interactions and it has always been my pleasure to confirm in words what the learning-disabled people they have met told them in 'pure human' – that they are good people. I have found it immensely satisfying to mentor students in nursing and social care situations with learning-disabled and autistic people. To meet these amazing personalities who are following a career working with minority groups struggling in society, warms my heart and helps me to believe in the good of human nature.

I have never known a learning-disabled person to get someone's personality wrong.

That first week at the hospital in September 1986, I found the residents natural and welcoming. They sensed I was 'different' and did not overload me. Slowly, I began to notice that they liked me. I cannot say how much this affected my self-esteem. I had never before been accepted unconditionally by anyone in my whole life and it was decidedly mind blowing. No one had ever taken the time to understand me. I formed the impression that learning-disabled people and I had a lot in common. I sensed then what I have come to understand now - learning disability, like autism, is a product of different sorts of neurology.

We shared a common life experience – we were all misunderstood and judged negatively for being ourselves. We shared paranoia and nervousness among people who could access the majority culture and affect our ability to be valued. We were outcasts, written off by authority at various times. We were naturally defensive of each other until proved trustworthy. In that week, I found a vocation that I still follow today. I work with people who are different. I have a way of taking in their unique lives and helping them move into a better space – physically, mentally and spiritually. I perform the roles of interpreter, problem solver and mentor. I put my own expertise of being staggeringly different from the norm and finding solutions to work in the service of helping them succeed. Read *Keep on Keeping On* for more information.

I had found my vocation in life and began a long apprenticeship with people - made possible through being employed to work in the learning disability sector in a structured, committed and purposeful way. Until then I had observed people, read what I could and tried to have a life with people. I had begun to make a few camera club and cycling club friends, but this job gave me more of a start in life with people than I could have imagined at the time.

Being autistic means I like to have a plan. I worked as a nursing assistant, an important role in the life of the people in the hospital. Nursing assistants were the people who carried out the care service and had the deepest relationships with residents. I noticed that how we behaved and communicated could make or ruin someone's day. Making someone's day was surprisingly simple yet profound, and went to the heart of the human condition. One needs to be a good person, motivated by love to start, then to have time to be with people, to listen, to share, to like them, to respect them and to show all these things in everything one does. Learning-disabled people cannot be fooled, although they are well practiced at hiding this and maintaining a front. They fear bad people, and through fear they will hold on to their insights and fears - a state of being which autistic people know well.

I wanted to make more of a difference in this work and decided that a qualification would be a positive step towards cementing a career and started to train as a nurse. The route to qualifying as a nurse suited my autistic ways of doing things. There was a course with a syllabus leading to a qualification. The route had been planned and set out.

I spent the summer of 1986 travelling to interviews. A whole new start in my chosen vocation appealed to me, and I wanted to go in a definite direction in a new place. Wales is a country I have liked for as long as I can remember - I love the landscape. I had two interviews in Wales and had two offers of a place, a good choice. The following January I would be off to live and work in Wales, but until I went I had no idea how unready I was and how much I had not developed. Today, I know this is a common autistic experience. We get to our early twenties and look similar to everyone else, but we do not have the same level of development.

As a rule of thumb I say our development is half our chronological age. However, we have the same number years of life experience as our peer group. This adds up to a lot of detailed knowledge, experience and memories, without the maturity and developmental framework to make all this work in an adult life. No matter how much we know, we come unstuck on our lack of a framework to cope with what comes at us in life. Our development is still fragmented and not joined up enough for where we need to be in order to cope. That was my situation in Wales. I was away from home with a job and a purpose, but lacking in all sorts of things which I did not know or understand until I needed that level of development.

I mentor students at this age – early twenties. I know how they are doing and use my experience to help them fill in the gaps. I help them to feel good about themselves and find autistic -riendly ways of living and getting on with life. I like it when a student has gained enough from me not to need me anymore. What I facilitate is not rocket science, but a back filling of knowledge, expertise and self-esteem delivered from one autistic person to another. They usually have enough to be getting on with after a few months, or even a couple of sessions if their requirements are very specific. A huge autistic advantage is our drive to get on with it once we know what progress is and how to do it.

In 1987 I knew I was in difficulties and had no idea why or what to do about it. I lacked the social and organisational skills to cope. I tried hard to make friends and get on with life - working until I was exhausted. I made it to July, then crashed in depression and feelings of suicide. I was making good progress – more than I thought – but when self-esteem is non-existent and confusion at life takes over, despair is not far behind. The killer problems were non-existent self-esteem allied with uncontrollable anxiety. How can an autistic person know if they are doing well if they are not told how to recognise and measure success? Remember - we autistics are told constantly that we are a problem through our lives, so it is natural that we build up negative understandings of who we are, which we believe deeply.

I did not know how to handle myself outside of doing job tasks. Undiagnosed dyslexia and the attendant organisational difficulties meant I was not handing in essays, despite learning very well and getting glowing placement reports. Charge nurses said I was one of the best students they had encountered and felt I had a good future in this work. Yet I sat at the desk in my room staring at the paper, writing very little, not even understanding the questions. Complete panic took over me as it did at school. I knew the subject well yet no words came.

Loneliness was also taking over. I had no idea how to live as a single person in nursing accommodation. Inside my head, I fought with pain and despair. Suicide attracted me every evening - a sweet end to the pain. I do not know how to describe the agony of a life falling apart. My ambitions seemed to be going nowhere.

An autistic person without hope for the future is in a bad way. We need a plan and to have detailed knowledge of how we can affect our lives for the better. In the absence of this knowledge we will rapidly decline into depression. I did not know it then, but I deliberately reach out with this lifeline of help regarding panic stations to young people I mentor now. I was young and had a lot of possible futures ahead, but I was following one plan and it was going wrong. I also had no idea of how to make things better, nor the ability to gather the strength to find help. Life became about survival – all hope had gone; I was in a panic.

I Dream In Autism

Panic is the condition of young autistic adults allied with despair. We have been told we are faulty up to this point by friends, family, teachers, employers – everyone we encounter is quick to point out how incoherent we are. We do not believe in ourselves and we know we are way behind people of our own age. The main thing I offer autistic people, especially young adults, is the benefit of my hindsight and help them to make plans. I form ways to cope, ways they can feel good about who and what they are, and help them see that they have a future. I show them they can change, make new plans and take their place in life. Hearing this from me helps, as they know I have been through it and come out the other side with success, relationships, a family and happiness. They see me as a reliable guide. I do my best.

What did help me though the dark times facing me was the support of the friends I had made who shared my obsessive interests (cycling and photography). They understood my differences and noticed I was struggling. I am very grateful to those wonderful people and have been for decades. There is a fresh openness about Welsh culture, something that attracted me to live in Wales along with the beautiful scenery. Lots of Welsh people will listen and share their lives openly - they certainly helped to save mine.

Being autistic, I sought a structure for socialising based round an interest. I found out about a local folk club and went for a drink. For a time, a group of us would meet up and I sought solace in those evenings at the folk club.

I also joined the Cardiff cycle club and became instantly confused by the culture of another cycle group after being a member of my local one for years. Being a university city, the Cardiff club had a younger membership profile. That was fine, however they wanted to ride shorter distances and stop at more pubs. That was fine too, I like a drink or two, enough to relax with and be able to talk. However, I could not place drinking into cycling. The two did not fit in my autistic understanding. The club I had ridden with previously rode all day, carried food and covered large distances in all weathers. That is called hard riding.

Eventually, I took myself out for solitary rides, long ones with food in my bag. But that did not work, as I hated being lonely. I cycle lots to get to different places or meetings but I have never been able to enjoy lone leisure cycling much. Cycling for me before then was my main social outlet.

Every change set me back. I realised I had no mechanism to accommodate changes. I was young and raw. Now I know that autistic people's social and emotional ages are half our chronological age. So back then I was a twenty one year old with the inner tool kit of a ten year old. No wonder I did not survive long. This is something I come across in my work a lot - young autistic adults leaving education with the expectation they will cope like their non-autistic age peers, but not being able to cope when they arrive in society.

 Like me, they can go into a deep depression and lose hope. The main thing I show them is that they are developing normally for an autistic person. That goes a long way to relieve their anxiety, but not entirely, as they are still behind their age peers and that is very hard to live with. Instead, we make a new plan based on their autistic development. We don't even start to round out until we have passed thirty. Some of us, me included, need to pass forty years old before rounding out developmentally. I can have fun with this today because that puts me in my early twenties again, but this time round I am mature, have a family and a successful career.

Back at twenty-one years old, I could not see a future beyond failure and depression. I knew I was worthy of a happy life but nothing else in my makeup matched that, so I kept failing – or so I saw it. In the summer months, I lost the will to be strong enough to carry on and one evening on the way back from work a colleague gave me a lift. I said how I felt and that I thought I was no good – I explained I had lost hope and wanted to leave the nursing course. That is where good friends can be a lot of help.

He said he thought I was doing well and was one of the best students in our intake. He was telling the truth, I knew it back then but could not internalise it because I felt so bad. It is the difference between knowing and believing something. I could believe nothing good about myself and had not for as long as I could remember. I had been programmed to accept I was worthless.

That evening I just had to do something, I had no idea what, but I needed to move. Movement has been my most frequently used stress reliever, normally cycling or just rocking and moving from room to room helps my anxiety levels if I am indoors. But that evening I got into my car and drove for miles. I had no place in mind, I just drove. As I put my foot on the accelerator and started to go faster the tears flowed down my face. There was little respite from moving. It was getting darker outside and I had neither plan nor hope. I wanted to die. Yet something in me would not let me crash the car into a bridge - there was a thread of life inside me making me go on. I turned onto the motorway and headed for my parents' house, the place I could stay with the highest chance of living.

What followed in the coming months was not good and I do not dwell on it too much. The darkness of depression is not something I want to write about. I have moved on. In those months, my parents and friends kept me alive. I had two very good friends in my home town. We used to go to the pub a lot where I would drink, talk and gain some respite from the darkness of depression. My parents suffered a lot, I am sure, in this time but they gave me somewhere to live. Back in Wales I had more good friends whom I would visit regularly, driving long distances for the monotonous peace of an open road and going to the pub for release. Their encouragement and time to talk meant a lot. I figured that I must not be so bad after all if people cared about me and that was an external source of help that comforted the darkness inside.

I returned to the nursing course in the following January with just about enough strength to carry on. I so wanted to complete the course and have a career in nursing. I knew the good work I could do with being a qualified nurse and that distant hope drove me on. I managed to keep going until April that year, then crashed again, this time into a deeper depression, which needed in-patient care.

I was lucky to be where I was; in that area there were mental health services that were more forward looking and better than most. The care I had was based on getting me to do nothing. They made me stop and do nothing until I could begin to calm down. I did not like that at first, but after a few weeks I got the hang of doing less and thinking less allowing my mind and soul time to cool off.

Most of all, I liked the wood workshop in the hospital, and after a time of enforced inactivity I was shown the day services. I went straight for woodwork. I love making things. I lost myself for hours at a time in wood. I made a model car, quite large with lots of moving parts. Then a large model windmill with turning sails, and every detail I had time to make. I still have both of them.

While in hospital I made trips out to see family and friends. I was very pleased to see my best friends from home one day. It meant so much that people showed they liked me and cared. That alone did more for my recovery than anything else. I would reflect on this for hours, usually at night when I could not sleep.

I returned to the nursing course briefly that summer with all the strength I could muster, but for a third time things went wrong, I lost hope, became suicidal and resigned from the course. It was something I did with great sadness, but I could not see a way forward. In fact I had every chance of finishing the course with good marks, but when depressed and with no hope, I could not see that. I packed up my things and went back home. I felt despondent, but was constantly exhausted and had no strength to carry on. That was the start of my weeks of being unemployed. They were miserable. I wanted so much to do something, to have a direction. I tried suicide once more on a summer's day when no one was around.

I Dream In Autism

I survived and carried on, one sad day at a time, with help from my colleagues, my car - a Citroen 2CV (I have had more of them than any other car) - and cycling chums. My parents were very good to me when I crashed the 2CV - a complete write-off. They helped me buy another one. I needed something as a distraction and source of pleasure. It helped a lot.

I still miss the 2CV I crashed, it was the best one I had, a blue 1983 Special. If I had known what I knew a few years later I would have rebuilt it on another chassis.

In late August, my father said there was work at the factory he sold products for. I wanted to work, recalling my summer holiday jobs in a factory a few years earlier. I liked the cadence and repetition of factory life. That was the end of my unemployment. I took a trip into Oxford before starting and bought a camera, something for the pure joy of it. I can chart my life by the cameras I have owned and the pictures I take. That purchase was the start of my recovery.

I spent about six weeks filling bottles with all sorts of decorating products, liking the cool dark factory and having something physical to do, it was like being back in the woodwork room. One top tip for employing autistic people - we are good at niche jobs that no one else likes. We like time in our own company, as social forms of working cause us to get tired and can reduce our efficiency. In that factory, no one wanted to fill the paint stripper bottles. The paint stripper was on its own in a corner - the foreman had a hard time getting anyone to do that job.

He asked me one day and I went for it with some enthusiasm. I could work on my own, hear the radio and earn a bit of money. I filled thousands of paint stripper bottles in that dark quiet place all day long. I also found a better way of doing it and loading the pallet, both of which went down well. I studied the viscosity of the paint stripper and got good at setting the valve and timing the arrival of bottles to make the process a lot faster. The trouble with that was I became too efficient and would run out of paint stripper – having to go back into the rest of the factory while waiting for another delivery.

Learning-disabled people were still my focus. My mum spotted a job advertised in a local home and I went for it. I was lucky - the manager was someone who would take a chance on 'someone like me'. A top tip for finding jobs if you are autistic - look for places where alternative people work as they are more likely to take you on and continue to employ you when your autistic profile becomes apparent at work.

That autumn I worked with learning-disabled people outside of a hospital setting. I loved the job and my colleagues. They were a fabulous group of people. We knew that was a special time to work together, and a lot of us have kept in touch.

Another top tip is to look for somewhere with a good atmosphere and supportive staff team. You will stand a much better chance of succeeding in work. Being autistic means we do not have the social skills to cope with the politics of a nasty workplace. I was bound to be a constant target for ridicule.

I worked in this home for six years and was sad to leave, but I got a job in a day centre specifically for learning-disabled adults. I liked working with clients in structured planning sessions. I liked the range of activities and did a lot of work with men. My job was exempted under the sex discrimination act. In people work, most of the workforce are women, which can cause difficulties for men being cared for - particularly young men. My brief was to be a man working with men, to help them feel good about their manhood and to act and develop in male ways. Men in the service sought me out and we had invaluable times tackling confidence issues by encouraging 'man stuff', like rebelling by putting our feet on tables and leaving dirty mugs out. These clients experienced liberation by behaving in gender stereotypical way – which was habitually alien to them.

We challenged their thought processes by making things like a brick barbecue or showed them how to be useful to others via fixing items. I started using 'dude' vocabulary in a safe environment by watching sport on television to allow clients bond and build relationships amongst their male counterparts – something they had never experienced before and thrived at. We increased moods by using humorous 'male' observations, such as pointedly expressing our ignorance at colour coordinated furniture, curtains or cushions. We washed and fixed cars, mended tools and did lots of conservation work. It was an empowering process for vulnerable residents and they enjoyed the methods and activities with great success. Results showed in their ability to safeguard their decision making routines – feeling confident in choices. They showed pride in themselves and a capability to interact with other people. They felt valued.

I loved the conservation work, being outside under the sky. The work was carried out in local nature reserves with the designated ranger service. We chopped things down, cleared paths, had bonfires, drove around in crew cab pickups, got wet and muddy, had snowball fights and got tired doing lots of hard physical work to help empower broken spirits.

I sometimes felt waves of contempt (caused by the workplace politics) in my daily role. Nearly all of my colleagues were decent people, but a handful operated for their own peculiar ends and envisaged ways to put down people that disagreed with them. There were also gossips and sycophants. I fell prey to these people many times. Some of them talked behind my back and engineered bullying tactics, but I did not have the skills or understanding to cope with them, so consequently spent a few occasions wondering what had happened to cause upset. And it was always me that felt the pain of torment. I could never work out why people applied to work in a caring service if they couldn't give their heartfelt goodness to others.

Support came from credible contemporaries who knew I was being deliberately provoked, using my autism as a weakness to undermine my results. These insightful people helped me to carry on bringing empowerment into the lives of residents, but were afraid of the hierarchical systematic politics. One of them said to me that I was 'too honest for this place'. I had ideas that were proactive and the clients liked my working style. I had an understanding of them, which was uniquely valuable on the staff team. I am autistic. I knew it then, but had not been diagnosed. I did not have the confidence to tell people about my differences, but I think some people within the care sector had started to work it out as the information became more widely available in theory form via medical research scientists.

There were several residents suffering from autism in the service where I worked. I could align myself naturally with them and help by 'walking the walk'. All my intuitive suggestions for client progression were accurate and acted upon. I recall a conversation with a psychologist about a client who needed to be approached extremely sensitively. I was their key worker for this situation and the psychologist said the plans I had drawn up for that particular clients' programme were completely beneficial; she had nothing to add.

I found that I could perform this type of care work naturally, but noticed that it would consequently annoy a manager who thought they knew everything about autism and how to handle the incoming cases. Autism was becoming more accepted, and, as I moved into my mid-twenties, instant experts appeared within the health care system, full of theories and academic approaches. Being an autistic sufferer, I could consistently deliver positive results in a more efficient and less conformist manner than the managers armed with textbooks and infographics. I confused many of the administrative powers by gaining success after success without the need for once referencing their unproved 'wisdom'.

Autistic clients are made for me. Their parents and carers confirm this by saying how pleased they are with the work I do - especially the understanding and advice I offer. I do not use what I call a 'system approach' to autism. I know the intricacies and inner world of autism better than anyone. You can see how it would upset someone in middle management who had been 'trained' to deal with the syndrome of autism, or those who appeared without a clue of what it feels like to live 24/7 within this state, but have a qualification in it – and expected to tell me how to do my job. My results proved that putting someone alongside the client who could behave in the same way and explain how to process anxiety was far more productive than their coloured flashcards or tight locking hugs to control meltdowns with physical embraces.

After some time, I won a dispute with the manager over my job grading and managed to earn some recognition for the success of my efforts – all with the support of the head of the service. This was a results-driven response for my autism client care. However, not long after this acknowledgement, the manager of the home made me redundant and I learned of the lengths people will go to if they let their pride rule over the best outcomes for clients. I was a threat to their system and had to go.

I watched the next professional assigned to the task arrive with interest – they were supposedly an autism expert but behaved with absolute ignorance for all things autistic. And this inexperienced, overqualified non-autistic person made mistake after irreparable mistake with the lives of people spiralling into depression. I was devastated, as I am normally seen as an asset in this line of care, but the administrative powers wanted things done their way. Within a few months, I was redeployed to another learning disability service nearer home and enjoyed a period of understanding compassion from the more senior people in the organisation that knew I was a useful asset with autistic sufferers.

In the new placement, I saw again that autism was not being understood, except via the use of reference books. I tried to step back and let them get on with it but eventually became involved through natural interaction. My comments and suggestions were noted as useful. Some were put into practise and after a few months of certain progressive outcomes involving disruptive and distressing residents, a manager asked me to set up and run the autism specialism in the service.

I had my dream job.

I set things up in ways that are unusual for an autism service. For a start, it did not look like an autism service provider at all. I knew the model being used in many services at that time was not tuned in to the sensitivities of autistic people.

Having an eclectic attitude to interventions and communication, my priority was to find people's places of comfort within communication and service culture. Luckily, my manager at this point was aware of my results and gave me full support. I wanted to supply a bespoke service – to see and treat each client as an individual, not as a syndrome. If a client needed colourful pictures and structured routines they had them, if not they did not. I used the 'what works best for each person' approach and became committed to person-centred working.

I was keen not to have a physically separate service, but the chance for space and quiet in a place serving the people who needed it most meant a designated room became made available for those who needed space. I majored on making the whole service autistic-friendly not autism theory. This involved staff training, development and lots of time from me explaining autism as a condition that can be celebrated and how we approach life with imbalanced cognitive ability for processing the things that non-autistics do instinctively.

A lot of what I taught seemed counter intuitive to a lot of people who saw autism as a behavioural problem, 'autistics don't feel empathy' and other such idiocy. We don't understand how to process emotions, but we do feel hurt by stupid ignorance and judgement just like everyone else.

I decided to show my skills in action. I had a client that I key worked with who had presented behavioural difficulties constantly throughout his life. His behaviour was caused and reinforced by working approaches over the years that saw this person as someone to be told off and fixed behaviourally. I asked a colleague, who was keen on what I was doing, to co-work my approach to the client. I needed something that would show people the efficacy of the ways of working I taught. I reckoned positive results of my philosophy would convince people. So we worked on helping the person feel good and reduce his stress. This was done simply by taking him as he was and trying to fix nothing.

We helped him restore his self-esteem. We checked out his physical health to see if there was anything physical he needed help with. A speech and language therapist found an eating difficulty. The result was the removal of high-risk food from his diet, leaving him all the things he liked anyway. He knew he had a swallowing difficulty but could not tell anyone, so he liked having this taken seriously and to have the problem solved. That, and the way we worked with him, was a turning point in his life. All the negative behaviours that gave concern stopped when he felt good about himself and less anxious.

From then on, the ways of working I developed gained traction, as the staff team saw good results for more people. It was lovely to see the view that autism was a behavioural issue go and be replaced with the view that autistic people are fine as they are. People became enthusiastic about the work I was doing and wanted to join in. Those were good days; I loved going to work.

Then, politics came in. I do not know why someone who is doing well cannot be appreciated. You see, the autism specialism I was running did not look like an autism specialism because I knew a more effective way of doing the work. I recall us calling in a consultant, who looked at the work we did. She said she could not suggest any improvements; she saw many comfortable autistic people and their comfort indicated that the right things were happening. I already knew that, but it was good to have it confirmed.

There were other ideas in the service about how autism work should be done. I knew about that, but believed that the results I was achieving spoke for the approach I designed. It was laid back and based on helping people find their place of comfort and natural means of communication. I set two success criteria for clients: one was that they were breathing and two, was that they had a pulse. This sent clients a powerful message - they are good enough just as they are, nothing needs to be fixed and no behaviour needs to be corrected.

Clients responded quickly to this approach. It was the first time in many of their lives they had not been seen as a problem to be fixed. I used my own experience to communicate the feeling very strongly that to be autistic is fine. What is needed is confidence, self-esteem and advice on how to get on in a non-autistic world. I knew these people had been challenged very strongly and often wrongly in their lives. They were survivors hence the two success criteria I set. I take the view that challenging behaviour is a form of communication used by people who are desperately unhappy and have no other option.

I knew it was felt elsewhere in the organisation that my methods were slack and the clients needed more rigour and structure in their service. Being autistic, I was unable to deal with the politics and hang around decision makers putting my case forward for argument. Gradually, I became aware the organisation was favouring the structured and what I call a 'tertiary approach', because it does not get to the heart of autism and does not see an autistic's personal inner world. I did... but few people would listen, except the clients and colleagues I worked with. Autism was well and truly on the map in medical terms with established rules designed by non-autistic people.

Over time, I was pushed sideways, and into a working pattern and environment where any autistic person could not be productive. I was getting a message that my services were not wanted any more, and cannot begin to say how much that hurt. The clients went back to being diagnosed as a condition – not treated as a person to be loved, mentored and monitored. I am autistic and know it inside out. I am widely read and very experienced in the work, with a huge record of success. But where politics are concerned, that does not count. Politics is something that is wholly outside the mode of operation of an autistic person.

I was made to work in an office under flickering tube lighting, with buzzers going off all day. Of course my mental health worsened. I was off with work-induced stress for extended periods of time. I melted down at work regularly through sensory overload, pain and anxiety. This was adding injury to insult – along with the added stress of seeing clients become anxious from being told what was best for them.

I started to wonder if I could work in the autism field as a freelance trainer and consultant and began my business www.autismlivetraining.com, using evenings and annual leave to establish my style of work. I am very good at what I do. People will call me in all to help with their caseloads across the UK. I am even able to travel abroad (fees paid by client) as my costs are minute compared to a large council or health service department with budgets and targets. I achieve results that save these institutions a great deal of time – and time costs money. I was told that my mentoring, service development and training skills were definitely worth something and I am very proud that this has become my life's work. I now go out into the world using my experiences, training and unique ability to convey the heart of autism from an autistic person to autistic users.

My business logo does not include a puzzle piece because, for me, autism is no mystery or puzzle to be solved - it is the stuff of my life and of those I work for. I am designed to be alongside autistic adults showing them how life can be something worth living. The more time I spent working in my freelance consulting business, the more in demand I became. So, I changed my hours to part time at my 'real job', because of my success rate, and eventually gave it up to work for myself full time. It was a very strange period in my life - in one job I was being sidelined and maltreated, and in the other I was welcome, wanted and in demand on my terms.

Working

When voluntary redundancies came up at work I applied, knowing exactly where my future was. For the first time I had a career of my own that I could grow. Since going freelance full time, I have never looked back and have enjoyed every bit of it. I am as good as my results.

I work as a consultant with the following incredible organisations: www.autismoxford.co.uk, www.faiersassociates.co.uk and www.seestheday.org.uk. These are businesses where I train and mentor in the world of autism. I get busier and busier, with humbling and happy results. Out in the world of freelance, as an autistic training consultant for autism service users, or family mentor, or 1:2:1 counselling, I only get business by being good at what I do and the results prove that.

I keep recalling the words of Temple Grandin when advising young autistic people about finding work. She said 'be super good at what you are good at'. That is sound advice and I repeat often. It is our strengths that get us work and on in life.

Autistic people are unable to cover up and use social skills to get on like non-autistic people can. We have to be on our mettle and be excellent at what we do. We are also good at niche work and the things other people do not like doing if we want to be embedded in the mainstream world - that gives us limited niches where we can work, do what we are good at and be happy.

275

Wandering And Ranging

I have always wanted to be on the move. However, I can be still if there is something interesting that will engage my intellect (even though my mind is still wandering). This mental behaviour often gets translated into physical wandering. I think when I move and I feel comfort when I move. I hold things in my consciousness and work on them when moving.

Right now, for sensory reasons, I have got to break off from my writing and clean up the dust around me. I will keep on working on this chapter and type it when I can get back to the computer. After twenty-five minutes of cleaning and sorting, putting the rubbish out and making a sandwich, I can get back to writing again. The dust is clear in my workspace and there is less to annoy my senses.

I have been on the move right round the house. I have checked the positions and condition of lots of things. I have refreshed my memory about home and where things are. I have repaired several gestalt models (thinking matrix – see 'Letter to a Mother') for accessing our house and finding things. The gestalt for this writing has come to the fore again. However my internet connection is down and I am sorting that out at the same time as writing. I want to listen to a BBC Radio 5 Live programme about troubled young people, ADHD and dyslexia, but the internet connection does not allow it, so as my brain is on form and what I call 'quick and slick'. I have to get going as it won't last long.

I have fixed the internet and loaded a film into a classic camera. My mind does go all over the place - I don't know what will be next. My mind wanders and I wander.

When I have not wandered for a while I get restless and grumpy. I have just been through winter - I don't wander far from home in winter. It has a lot to do with limited daylight. I am mentally planning to wander a lot more in the spring and summer. In the evenings, I surf the internet to find places to go in my mind and also with my family. I look on Flickr for pictures of places and

YouTube for videos of the same places. I go there in my mind and anticipate going there for real. I plan and plan and plan. This keeps me going thought the winter nights. I have booked a week off work for late March, after the clocks go forward for British Summer-time from GMT (Greenwich Mean Time). I will wander then. I have a small car and a folding bicycle to go exploring with.

I go to places that resonate with my interests and have memories attached. I like most places in Wales, anywhere in the Pennines and Cornwall, and several places on the coast, especially the north east of England. I go where there is water, sea, lakes or rivers. It's a good blessing for me, living on an island.

Nearer home, I wander on my bicycle or on foot. I go to places I know well. I photograph them and have built up a series of pictures showing these places over the last twenty or more years. I look at the pictures regularly. I like wildlife and love seeing which species will do well each year - the natural cycle of wildlife goes like that. Some species of plants and animals have particularly successful years but deplete their food sources. In succeeding years, they do less well and other species come to the fore, thus maintaining a balance, it's all wonderfully self-regulating. I take immense comfort in seeing this cycle.

I have been wandering for two weeks since I wrote these last words. I went downstairs to see to the washing machine, got into something else and have been busy on all sorts of stuff. I meant only to have a walk around the house and get back to writing, but instead, became distracted. This always happens – I have a lively mind and no organisation. I was exactly the same at school – I could not coordinate my studies, but I was bright minded. If the lessons were taken outside, I could have concentrated much easier. This is one of the tactics I use when mentoring. I walk with clients in the open countryside and work on interactions with them via this practise. We discuss plans and programmes. It is an incredibly effective communication tool – to hardly communicate at all. So, I have been meaning to get back to this writing on many occasions. I have also been thinking at night about what to write, but on getting up I do something completely different instead like tidying, dump runs, gardening, shopping, photography, enjoying springtime, fixing things, cycling, and going to see my parents. Today is the first day I could write. I have been so busy at work that it has taken me six days to get enough coherent thoughts together to write.

When I have a week off like this I usually go somewhere for a day in my car and travel some distance. This is a form of wandering I love. I will plan to go somewhere - the sea, the Welsh borders, or somewhere completely wild. I go to clear my head and feel peace in my soul. These wanderings are important. I do them two or three times a year. I take my folding bicycle and go riding far and wide. I love to have the wind in my hair, riding through beautiful, wild and ancient places. I explore the history of places and feel connected with life. No one can make a claim on me and I feel free, unjudged... whole again.

The long drives to these places are times for head clearing and peace. The displacement activity of driving helps me be still in my head. The vision of green countryside going past soothes my sight. My car is a peaceful machine. It is quiet, unassuming, the controls are light, smooth and predictable, they sooth my sensory experience. The engine is low powered and just purrs along, it does not need to be revved, nor do gears need changing often. The whole experience is soothing. My car is also very well built, good for sensory reasons. It is fourteen years old and is as clean and tight as a three-year-old car, a combination of good build quality and meticulous maintenance.

Six months has passed and I am back at this piece of writing. I have thought a lot in the meantime. Writing all this down has taken years of dedication, so I write what I can when I can. My editor is keen for me to keep my voice, passion and professionalism in this text. She is aware that the message of autism must be felt through my expressions. Apologies if I repeat or annoy – it is part of my makeup. I am obsessed with cameras and bicycles and engineering feats, large or small, so want to relay this with you – to make sure you understand how an autistic person thinks. Remember this… please remember what I have told you when you meet one of us and are asked over and over again to listen to us about an interest. I have my tale to tell and use it to let parents see what their children are feeling. I often find ways to communicate with client siblings, or loved ones trapped in their own autistic world, by looking back at my experiences and talking through the thoughts and feelings I had. This book is meant to be picked up and put down. To be mused and used.

So, as I was telling you… I escape through my bicycles. They are high quality and well-designed machines. Two are fully suspended for road use. I go miles on them. I get fit, breathe deeply, burn adrenaline and wander in my mind to far-off places and times. I listen to the purr of the tyres and the rustle of the chain. These are moderated by the up and down of my legs, causing these sounds to interweave. I have to keep telling you this because I am autistic. Do you recognise this trait in people you know?

I have always had the need to wander and find peace. On family holidays I would seek out peaceful places to go. Before I started school, we stayed at a holiday bungalow in Slade on the Gower Peninsula. I would go outside with my toy cars and become immersed in a world of cars, sky, pure thinking and happiness. I watched the clouds, felt the wind on my face, stared at trees – counting their leaves, watched birds flap wings against their chest, listened to the sound of cattle and the distant sea. I would become utterly wrapped up in all of this information - completely lost in a reverie of daydreams. It was a place of sweet happiness. Then I would be called in, for meals or to join in some event inside. These times troubled me because my peace was broken. People moved around me in a blur, they spoke a lot - I became anxious and did not follow their meanings. I recall my name being called on occasions, again and again. Such was my giddy incomprehension that I responded only after my name was called several times. I heard comments like 'he's always like that' or 'dilly daydream'. It was as if, when surrounded by people, I existed in a giddy world of half heard, half seen people who sometimes stopped long enough for me to perceive them clearly.

The best times on that holiday were when we were out on the beach, or where there were rocks, on the way round the coast to Horton. These rocks had deep ridges in them. I recall running from ridge to ridge with young friends from the family with whom we were sharing the holiday bungalow. We would be characters from the Magic Roundabout. I was Dougal. I remember singing 'I'm a Dougal, I'm a Dougal' in time with my footsteps on the rocks. It was the last time I can remember feeling completely at peace – before I started school and the bullying happened. I recall the sunshine up above, the shiny sea, and my friends running in the sunlight.

Every time I hear Debussy's 'Images for the Piano' I am transported back to those sunny, silver days on the rocks by Slade. I go straight back to the feelings I felt in that space – and revisit this memory on most days. It's like a precious talisman that I get out when life hurts. I was free and happy when standing so young full of life on the rocks at Slade. The memory carries stillness and happiness that I can access at any time. The Dalai Lama says 'it is a miracle we are born at all – what will you do with your life?'. I am at peace with mine now, but it took decades of pain to get here. I know I am on this earth to help others who are suffering as I did. Autism Live Training is exactly that – autism living alongside autism.

Nowadays, I stand by the sea, lost in waves, foam, wind and natural sounds. I am happy in my own skin. I am me. If I cannot get to the sea, I do this in my head, I have many videos with sound I can play and lose my whole self in. I play music and lose myself there too. I can wander and be still if I can go on travels in my head.

On my bicycle, I ride along lanes and lose myself in the passing tarmac and hedgerows. It is here that real thinking and coordination happens. My bicycle must be in perfect working order, so any imperfections do not drown out my thoughts.

I Dream In Autism

Moving freely, I feel alive and have done for as long as I remember. When I was young I had a tricycle and a pedal car. They were my treasures; I could move freely on them, get to otherwise unattainable speeds, feel the rush of wind on my face and arms, feel them moving over the ground, feel them going up and down over slopes and bumps, feel the wheels frame and steering working. These treasures were added to my body for freedom and speed as I have always walked awkwardly and hurt my feet on the ground. Now I know I have a poor sense of my body, my leg length and reflexes are uncoordinated. Walking is uncomfortable, but I do walk a lot as walking can get me to places that wheels cannot. Walking enables wandering, especially when I have our dog with me. Walking gets me up hills, on paths, over cliffs, rocks, streams, heather, sand dunes and up to views that are beautiful beyond words.

Yet being on a bicycle is wandering heaven. Spinning wheels, wind on my face and the rush of movement is the place I want to be. I teach the saying that to travel hopefully is a better thing than to arrive. Remember that I am autistic, so I take this saying literally and do not mean it in the way most people take it. There is nothing about hope and ambition in my interpretation - I literally mean the physical journey. Being autistic, interactions with people at the end of the journey can be uncertain; travel is simple and calm.

I am getting better in later life at arriving and dealing with people, but as a child the journey was all. When at the destination, I lived for the journey home. Today I can look forward to having a fully valued working life at the other end of the journey. I am actually helping people. I have learned enough scripts and forms for this and to be able to enjoy people's company freely on arrival. That is so good.

-ENDS-

Printed in Great Britain
by Amazon